FORBIDDEN ALCHEMY

TRANSMUTING TABOO INTO EROTIC MEDICINE

SHARON MARIE SCOTT

Forbidden Alchemy: Transmuting Taboo into Erotic Medicine

Edited by Lexi Mohney and Anna Paradox
Cover Design by Kristina Edstrom

An Imprint for GracePoint Publishing
(www.GracePointPublishing.com)

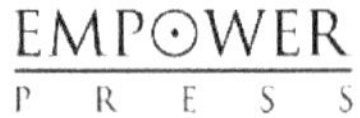

GracePoint Matrix, LLC
624 S. Cascade Ave, Suite 201
Colorado Springs, CO 80903
www.GracePointMatrix.com
Email: Admin@GracePointMatrix.com
SAN # 991-6032

A Library of Congress Control Number has been requested and is pending.

ISBN (Paperback): 978-1-966346-67-8
eISBN: 978-1-966346-68-5

Books may be purchased for educational, business, or sales promotional use.
For distribution queries contact Sales@IPGbook.com
For non-retail bulk order requests contact Orders@GracePointPublishing.com

Printed in U.S.A

CONTENT WARNING

This book contains mature content intended for adult readers.

The author explores sexuality, power dynamics, and alternative relationship structures with unflinching honesty. This work is designed to challenge cultural taboos and examine the intersection of eroticism and spirituality.

This book contains sexually explicit language, detailed descriptions of sexual experiences, BDSM practices, power exchange dynamics, and consensual non-consent scenarios. It also explores childhood trauma, emotional wounds, codependency, and challenges to conventional religious frameworks.

This book is an invitation to examine what you've been taught to fear about your own desires. It does not prescribe a particular path, nor does it claim that these experiences are universal or necessary. Rather, it offers one person's journey through the edges of cultural taboo toward personal sovereignty and erotic wholeness.

All experiences and practices described involve informed consent between adults. This work advocates for awareness, communication, and personal agency in all intimate exchanges.

If you choose to engage with this material, do so with self-awareness and respect for your own boundaries.

LOOK FOR THESE OTHER WORKS BY SHARON MARIE SCOTT

COMICS

More Than Mortal
More Than Mortal: Truths & Legends
More Than Mortal: Sagas
More Than Mortal: A Legend Reborn
The Witchfinder
Lady Pendragon/More Than Mortal crossover
Makebelieve
Alien Confidential (web comic)
Illuminati: Out of Chaos Comes Order

FICTION

The Secret Letter Society
Project Orion (novel, content Developer + producer)
Write Now! Science Fiction, Fantasy, and Horror (contributing author - *Writing the Genre Series)*

GAMES AND COLLECTIBLES

Young Justice: Legacy (video game)
Falling Skies (video game)
Outlander (collectible trading card set, seasons 1-3)
Barbie: Groom and Glam Pups (video game)
Barbie: Jet, Set, and Style (video game)
Sherlock Holmes Mysteries (mobile game)
Castle (board game)
Po's Kung Fu Challenge (mobile game)
Planes: Fire and Rescue video game (mobile game)
Unsung Story (video game)
Busy Scissors (video game)
Dr. Cockroach's Monster Generator (mobile game)
Max Steel Online (video game)

FILM

Mistborn Trilogy (film treatments)

To every part of me that was told her desire was dangerous.

To the alchemy that turned shame into fire.

And to everyone daring to make the forbidden sacred again—this book is for you.

CONTENTS

PART FIVE: THE FINAL EDGE
PLEASURE AS SPIRITUAL MASTERY

INTRODUCTION

This book is an act of rebellion—and reverence. A spell woven in ink. Not because I set out to write a "kink book" (though it is full of sex, power, and desire), but because taboo has always been my teacher. Every time I've peeled back the layers of conditioning—about sex and relationships, about power, or about spirituality—I've found something sacred underneath. Not a God of rules, but a divine, radiant Source within that insists on being experienced through the body.

I was raised to be small. To behave. To *never embarrass the family* with my curiosity or my wildness. But something in me always asked: What else is there?

When I stopped silencing that voice, everything changed.

I learned to hold what once felt like opposites—pleasure and reverence, grief and intimacy, rage and devotion—and discovered that together they didn't cancel each other out. They made life feel *more alive*.

FROM FEAR TO FREEDOM: THE JOURNEY AHEAD

Here's what I've discovered:

Fear is the first cage. It keeps us compliant. Afraid to want, afraid to feel, afraid to lose love.

From fear, we drop into *need*—the survival impulse. The place where we contort ourselves to get just enough to stay alive.

But beneath need waits *desire*—raw and beautiful. Unapologetic.

And just before we touch that desire? We often meet *shame*. Not as a stop sign, but as a signal: *You're approaching something powerful.* Shame is what we've been taught to feel when we near our truth.

When you can hold desire *without collapsing into shame,* you unlock *choice*. Real choice. Not the kind that comes from reaction or fear of rejection. The kind that comes from sovereignty.

Forbidden Alchemy stands at that threshold between shame and choice.

WHAT THIS BOOK IS (AND ISN'T)

This isn't an encyclopedia of kink or a manual of techniques.

What you'll find here are stories:

- My own lived thresholds.
- Moments I witnessed in my communities.
- Memories entrusted to me by people I love and respect.

Each reveals something about the edges we fear and the way those edges hold medicine.

You'll meet the paradox of power in different forms: how submission can be a portal to sovereignty, how surrender can lead to ultimate control, how wielding power as a Dominant can deepen intimacy rather than create distance. You'll explore the spectrum of the taboo and the exquisite balance of opposites—Dominant/submissive, Top/bottom, Daddy Dom/baby girl, Primal Predator/Prey, Exhibitionist/Voyeur, and beyond.

If you have been waiting for permission, this is it.

You don't have to hold back anymore. Or shrink. You don't have to deny the parts of yourself that scare you.

This book is a *summoning.* The edge has already been calling you. It always has.

This is where alchemy happens—where the very desires you were taught to fear become the blueprint for your freedom and self-mastery.

THE MEDICINE OF PLEASURE

Pleasure isn't just a sensation. **Pleasure is a technology**.

It is an advanced system of vibrational expansion, a mechanism for dissolving illusions, and an energetic force that—when wielded consciously—has the power to rewire everything—your thoughts and emotions, your physical form… even the reality you live in.

The world has tried to convince you that pleasure is indulgent. That it must be controlled and rationed, or denied entirely. But when a person fully owns their pleasure, *something shifts.* You stop waiting to be told what you're allowed to feel. Which means you become *ungovernable.*

A NOTE ON LANGUAGE

Because this book is rooted in alternative lifestyles and power exchange, language matters. A single word, a capital letter, a pronoun—each carries a charge. Here's how I use them.

Three words frame this book:

- Taboo. The edges of culture—the places we're told to fear. Sex, rage, pleasure, power, grief, hunger, God. Taboo isn't evil. It's forbidden. *Which means it's sacred.*
- Erotic. Not pornography or performance. The Erotic is life-force. The shiver when truth hits, the ache of wanting, the pulse that reminds you you're alive.
- Medicine. Not to fix, but to reveal. Medicine is the alchemy that turns shame into power and fear into desire.

Capitalization & Roles:

- Domme/Dominant/Top are capitalized, as are pronouns referring to them (He, She, They). Not because they're "above," but to mark chosen authority.
- submissive/sub/bottom stays lowercase. Again—not diminishment. A chosen polarity.
- Archetypal forces like Dark Feminine and Dark Masculine are capitalized because they are energetic currents, not personal traits.

Dirty Words, Reclaimed:

For centuries, words like *pussy*, *slut*, *fuck*, and *cock* have been twisted into insults or stripped of reverence. In these pages, they return to their rightful place. For me, that means sacred and potent.

- When I write *pussy*, it's worship, not diminishment.
- When I call myself a *slut*, it's reclamation: hunger owned without apology.
- When I say *fuck*, it's not vulgar—it's raw intensity.
- When I write *cock*, it's not a joke—it's reverence for the power and presence of arousal itself.

If these words make you pause, good. Let them. They're spells meant to show you where your edges are.

THE INVITATION

This isn't a book to consume passively. It's a mirror. An initiation. An invitation to meet the parts of yourself you've been told were too much, too strange, or too forbidden—and discover the power that was waiting there all along.

Your edges guide you.

Your pleasure fuels you.

Let's begin.

PART ONE: INITIATION

THE ALCHEMY OF DESIRE

CHAPTER 1

THE DARK FEMININE & THE DARK MASCULINE

Maybe you've felt it before. That yearning in your body you can't explain but can't ignore. A craving for a partner who'll take the lead so you can finally let go. A hunger for someone so fierce that it consumes you. Or maybe it's the surge in you that wants to step up and take control. The urge to break every rule and let yourself go wild.

Those longings aren't random. They're how the Dark Feminine and the Dark Masculine move through you.

They aren't gendered roles—they're currents, energetic forces that live in each of us.

Culture taught us to fear these parts of ourselves because they don't play by the rules or obey propriety. They don't keep us small or polite or manageable. And so, especially in women and *especially in our sexuality,* they were buried.

But they never left. They are primal truths. You only forgot.

Like other archetypes, the Dark Feminine and the Dark Masculine show up in two ways: distortion and coherence. What some traditions call "shadow," I'll often call distortion. Not because the energy itself is bad—but because it's out of alignment, out of coherence. And here's the key: Every distortion carries the seed of a gift. The boss who crushed your ideas is the distorted face of the same energy that, in coherence, becomes unwavering leadership. The lover who twists your words to get their way is the distorted face of the same energy that, in coherence, looks you in the eye and speaks the hard truth.

So the point isn't to reject these dark currents. It's to learn how to recognize them—first in distortion, then in coherence—so their real power can move through you.

SIDEBAR: Light and Dark

When I use the words Light and Dark in this book, I don't mean "good" and "bad." These aren't moral labels. Light describes the qualities most people are already familiar with in Masculine and Feminine energies: order, harmony, receptivity, expression. Dark points to the edges we're less comfortable naming—intensity, power, destruction, surrender, ecstasy, annihilation. The Light soothes. The Dark transforms. Both are sacred currents, and both belong in our erotic and spiritual wholeness.

THE DARK FEMININE

The Dark Feminine is the current that dissolves. That devours. That births. It's the hunger that won't be silenced. It's the chaos that tears down what isn't real. The primal force that pulls you into the unknown.

In distortion, the Dark Feminine can be manipulative, destructive, and consuming. Maybe you've seen it in yourself in moments of jealousy or rage, or a neediness that took you over. You might've seen it in a partner who withholds affection to keep you chasing them, or in the parent who guilt-trips in order to control.

But in coherence, the Dark Feminine is liberation itself. She's the voice in you that finally says, *I can't keep living like this.* She's the one that quits the job that's killing her spirit, ends the relationship that's draining her soul, or finally says the thing everyone else is afraid to say. She's the one who chooses aliveness even when it costs everything—that's the Dark Feminine: dissolution, desire, the force that strips you bare and births you anew.

THE DARK MASCULINE

The Dark Masculine is the current that grips. That holds. That cuts through. It's the part of you that sets a boundary and won't back down. The presence that stays steady no matter how many wildfires are burning around you. The discipline that pushes you past your excuses to find the strength you didn't know you had.

In distortion, the Dark Masculine can become rigid or controlling, even cruel. Maybe you've felt that in yourself too, when your need to control squeezes the life out of something. Or in others—a parent who told you you'd never succeed, the friend who always had to win, or the partner who turned intimacy into a power game.

But in coherence, the Dark Masculine is the cleanest container you'll ever know. The coach who demanded your best and made you proud you didn't quit. The lover whose steady, unshakable presence let you open to more pleasure than you thought was possible. Or the fire in you that refuses to back down until the work is done—that's the Dark Masculine in coherence: structure, direction, unshakable presence.

TOGETHER

If the Dark Masculine stands firm without the Dark Feminine, nothing ever changes. If the Dark Feminine tears through without the Dark Masculine, everything collapses into chaos. But when they meet—when one holds steady while the other breaks through—that's when something new can be born.

The Dark Masculine holds. The Dark Feminine breaks through. One is the pillar that doesn't waver. The other strips away the false so truth can rise. Together, they create the pressure that births expansion.

MYTHIC RESONANCE

These currents have been in our stories forever.

The Dark Feminine rises first: Lilith, the first wife of Adam, refuses to bow—she is the defiant voice that says, *I will not shrink to be loved.* Kali, Hindu goddess of destruction and liberation, draped in skulls, devours illusion with wild laughter until nothing remains but raw truth. Medusa, the serpent-haired Gorgon, stops pretense in its tracks—her gaze the mirror that forces you to face what you'd rather deny.

And then the Dark Masculine: Ares, god of war, charges forward with uncompromising force—the embodiment of raw drive and direction. Shiva, the ascetic and yogi, sits unmoving in meditation—his stillness the vast container that holds the cosmos itself. Osiris, judge of the underworld, weighs every heart against the feather of truth—structure, law, and exactness embodied.

These figures aren't just old myths. They're reminders that the Dark Feminine and Dark Masculine have always lived in us. We didn't invent them—and they never left.

You'll feel these currents most vividly in the erotic body: when pleasure builds until you think you can't take more—your breath stutters, your muscles tense—yet something in you keeps going. That's where the medicine lives. At the edge, pleasure isn't just sensation. It's the fire that burns away old wounds. It's the opening that lets your spirit expand. It's the moment your body reclaims what you were once told to bury.

What once felt like *too much* is exactly what sets you free.

You'll meet these currents again and again in the chapters ahead—in kink, in devotion, in primal play, in relationship. They'll rise in every taboo you've hidden and every edge that secretly turns you on.

Now you have names for them. Now you can feel them for what they are.

And from here—we play.

EROTIC ALCHEMY IN PRACTICE: MEETING THE CURRENTS

Embodiment

Recall a recent moment when you felt restless or frustrated—hungry for something. Notice how your body carries the charge of that moment—maybe your breath quickens, your jaw clenches, heat rises in your chest. This is one way your Dark Feminine shows up: raw, demanding, unwilling to stay quiet.

Now recall a moment when you felt grounded and unshakable. Notice those signals: maybe your shoulders drop, your breath slows, your spine straightens. This is one way your Dark Masculine shows up: steady, present, unmovable.

> **Spicy Add-On:** Bring touch into it. Use one hand to claw or squeeze or scratch your body as your Dark Feminine voice rises. Then switch—press the other hand firmly on your chest, your thigh, your hip as your Dark Masculine holds steady. Let your arousal build as the two currents clash and merge.

Expression

On paper, let these two voices speak. Let your Dark Feminine say what she wants, or what she refuses to silence. Then let the Dark Masculine respond—let him state what he offers, how he steadies, or what he promises to hold. Go back and forth without editing.

> **Spicy Add-On:** If you want to take it further, speak the dialogue out loud in front of a mirror. Let your body

move with each voice: hips circling, voice raised, chest heaving for the Feminine; shoulders squaring, tone dropping, feet grounding for the Masculine. Watch yourself embody both.

Spicier Add-On: If you want to push this further, share your notes with someone you trust. Read aloud a line from your Dark Feminine, then let them embody the Dark Masculine by simply responding with steady presence: "I hear you. I can hold that."

Switch roles if it feels good.

Integration (24-Hour Challenge)

Over the next day, watch for when one of these energies rises in you. When the Dark Feminine flares—hungry, restless, or loud—ask: What is she really asking for? When the Dark Masculine rises—quiet, calm, anchored—ask: What is he protecting or holding steady for me? Let your choices in the moments after that reflect that awareness.

Spicy Add-On: Give the energy a place to land. When your Dark Feminine rises during the day, excuse yourself to the bathroom or bedroom and let her move—growl, grind against a pillow, or moan into your hand. When the Dark Masculine rises, ground it: Stand firm, grip the edge of a table, look at yourself in the mirror, and say, "I've got this."

CHAPTER 2

THE BLINDFOLD & THE UNKNOWN

SURRENDERING PERCEPTION, AWAKENING POWER

There's a moment, just before the fabric touches your skin, when the world still holds its shape. A moment when you can see what's coming, when you know the light is about to vanish, but you haven't yet surrendered to the dark.

And then—

The blindfold slides into place.

Your world collapses inward. The edges blur. What was once vast and full of detail becomes something else entirely:

Sensation.

Breath.

Heartbeat.

Presence.

In the absence of sight, something else awakens. Your awareness stretches beyond what you can see. Without the distraction of perception, you *feel more.*

This is the first gate: the moment the body stops relying on external cues and starts listening to something deeper. Something primal and divine.

The mind, so accustomed to logic and sight, hesitates at first, scanning the void, grasping for predictability. But the body? The body doesn't hesitate. The body knows. It doesn't need to be seen to understand. It listens, then responds and moves in the language of energy and sensation and instinct.

This is what so many forget—sight is not the only way to *know*. **The deeper truth lives in the body**. It's just waiting for us to surrender enough to feel it.

THE FIRST TIME I LET GO

The blindfold was one of my earliest entrances into kink. The first time I wore one, I expected darkness. I didn't expect the *space* it created.

The moment sight was gone, everything else surged forward: the heat of my own body. The brush of air across my arm, the sound of my own breath, louder than I'd ever heard. Without my eyes to track or anticipate, I couldn't escape into control. Every flicker of sensation landed sharper, fuller, inescapable.

And beneath it all, something shifted. I'd spent my whole life watching—scanning for approval, scanning for danger, scanning for permission. I had built an entire identity around being able to see *everything*, to anticipate others' needs and feelings, as a way to feel in control. But the blindfold... the blindfold stripped all of that away. For maybe the first time, I was *feeling myself* from the inside out.

The hand that tied the blindfold was the Dark Masculine current—structure, containment, presence. The catch of my breath and the heat that rose in me was the Dark Feminine—surrender, hunger, aliveness.

The blindfold wasn't just a prop. It was an initiation that whispered: *There is more here than you've been willing to feel.*

THE WISDOM IN THE DARK

In a world that demands certainty, the blindfold drags you into the unknown. It pulls you out of the mind's constant scanning and drops you into sensation and trust.

For those of us who have spent our lives bracing for impact or performing for approval, the dark can feel like relief. It's the permission we didn't know we needed to stop watching ourselves be watched, to stop managing, and simply *be.*

This is the real gift of the blindfold: not just the intensity of touch, but the shift back into presence. The power of no longer seeing yourself from the outside but feeling yourself fully from within.

The dark doesn't strip you of power—it reveals it. Without external perception weighing on you, you meet the raw currents inside: the Dark Feminine, who doesn't wait for permission to feel, and the Dark Masculine, who steadies her fire so it doesn't consume everything in its path.

This is the paradox of power: surrender held by structure. It's where pleasure sharpens into presence, and where the mystery of the unknown becomes the place you discover your own depth.

BEYOND THE BLINDFOLD: THE POWER OF SENSORY DEPRIVATION

The blindfold was my first introduction to sensory deprivation, but it wasn't the last. Sensory deprivation isn't just about blindfolds—it's about full immersion. When external stimuli are stripped away—hoods, earplugs, gags, bondage that restricts movement—imagination awakens.

This is why sensory deprivation is alive in both kink and mysticism. When there's nothing left to interpret or react to, you're left with only what's real inside you.

To surrender to that is the moment control drops away, and raw presence takes its place:

What happens when all there is to do is *be*?

CLOSING THE SCENE: TRUSTING THE UNKNOWN

Some truths only reveal themselves in the dark.

The blindfold isn't about losing something—it's about opening and no longer performing for what you think others see, so you start feeling what's actually alive in you.

This is the beginning. The first unraveling. Power not as control, but as presence. Pleasure as the compass that shows you where to go next.

The invitation? To let *the Mystery* have you. To stop bracing for what you know and allow the unknown to stir what's been asleep. Because the places you've avoided are often the very ones holding the power you've been searching for.

When you surrender perception, you don't get smaller—you expand. You remember your power, not through proof, but through the undeniable truth of sensation, of breath, and of presence.

EROTIC ALCHEMY IN PRACTICE: THE DARK INVITATION

Embodiment

Close your eyes or place a blindfold over them. Take a few slow breaths. Notice the shift when sight disappears. What feels different? Tune in to sound, to temperature, to the brush of air on your skin. Notice how sensation and presence become sharper when vision is gone.

> **Spicy Add-On:** Invite someone to guide you blindfolded across a room. Let them place different textures or objects for you to touch or step on as you go, or feed you small bites of food. Feel how disorienting and intimate it becomes to rely fully on their lead.

Integration—Solo

Play with everyday moments of sensory deprivation. Shower with your eyes closed. Eat a meal blindfolded. Explore self-pleasure in the dark, letting touch—not sight—be your guide. Let your Dark Feminine show you where she hungers to feel more, and let your Dark Masculine hold you safely with breath and presence.

> **Spicy Add-On:** Try self-pleasuring blindfolded with an unfamiliar object or texture (a feather, an ice cube, a toy you don't normally use). Let surprise itself become part of the arousal.

Integration—Partnered

Invite someone into a short blindfold scene. Let one of you wear the blindfold while the other offers simple, attentive touch—brushing fingertips across skin, breathing close to the ear, a piece of cloth dragged across the body. The one in the blindfold practices embodying the Dark Feminine current: surrendering into sensation. The one holding the space practices embodying the Dark Masculine current: presence without rush, containment without force.

Switch roles if desired.

> **Spicy Add-On:** Add a layer of suspense—let the one holding the space alternate between touch and deliberate pauses. The waiting becomes its own edge: not knowing when or where the next touch will land.

CHAPTER 3

BREAKING THROUGH

THE FIRST EDGE OF VISIBILITY & POWER

There are things we tell ourselves we are *not.* Not an exhibitionist. Not into pain. Not soft. Not wild. Not one of *those* people.

And then something happens—a moment, a crack in the foundation of the story you've built about yourself.

You can feel it before you can name it. That pull. That undeniable charge. That quiet knowing in the body, long before the mind will admit it.

The moment my Dominant put a leash on me, I felt the crack. The night I was led through the party and placed in a cage, I felt something in me shift.

But I told myself I wasn't one of *those* girls.

Not yet.

THE PARTY, THE CAGE, THE OPENING

There was magic in the hours just before our planned scene. A thick charge in the air, anticipation wrapping around my breath as I prepared. Tonight, I was to be on display.

I stepped into my strappy lingerie, the fabric whispering against my skin, soft against my hips and breasts, sending a shiver straight through me. The platform heels came next—sexy and statuesque. Powerful. A keystone of the night ahead. They made me feel both larger than life and utterly, beautifully small. As in *feminine*. Submissive. Desired.

The anticipation was a living thing inside me. I could feel it in my stomach, in the tightening of my chest, in the low, insistent warmth between my legs. I'd been collared before. I'd knelt before. I'd allowed myself to be led before.

But this was different.

Tonight, I wasn't just His. I was His to *show off.*

The leash around my neck tugged gently, a silent command, and I followed—not because I had to, but because part of me wanted to be marked in that way. To be led. To be claimed as a prize.

The air inside the dungeon was buzzing—leather and candle wax, the hum of conversation, the sound of impact play in more than one corner. Eyes followed us. I'd dressed to draw them—the eyes—and yet they felt like heat on my skin, an awareness prickling down my spine. Part of me wanted to shrink. To disappear into the dark corners of the room, where no one could see the flush rising on my cheeks. But I didn't.

I'd been in this space so many times before—peer-sharing and leading discussions—but never *like this*. Never in a position where I couldn't hide. He led me slowly, deliberately, guiding me with a sure hand, parading me in front of people as we made our way past various scenes of delightful torment: cock and ball torture, needles, electrical play...

And with every step, every set of lingering eyes, I felt myself sinking deeper into the collar and the scene, into submission, into *myself*. By the time we reached the cage, I was floating in the ether of it all, intoxicated by frequency alone.

The cage was narrow, but not so small that I couldn't kneel comfortably inside if I wanted to. The metal was cool against my exposed skin as I stepped in, my heart pounding in my chest. The door clicked shut behind me, the sound reverberating in my bones. My fingers curled around the bars, my body arching slightly as I settled into my place. Eyes tracked me—some curious, some amused, some filled with their own quiet hunger. There was nowhere to hide.

I gripped the bars tighter, knuckles white, my chest rising and falling as another flash of heat surged between my thighs. The cold metal pressed through the thin strappy fabric, sharp against my skin. My knees dug into the hard ground, my thighs trembling—not from strain, but from arousal I didn't want to admit.

A voice in the crowd laughed, another whispered, "Beautiful." The words ignited the very hunger I'd spent years trying to hide. My Dominant's hand brushed the bars near my face. He didn't touch me, but His presence steadied me while the rest of the room ate me alive with their eyes.

I was trapped. On display. *Seen.*

THE RUSH OF BEING WANTED, THE TERROR OF WANTING IT

A wave of arousal rushed through me, clashing violently against the familiar pulse of fear. The shame of being watched warred with something deeper, something hotter.

I wasn't supposed to *like this*. And yet...

There is an energetic shift that happens the moment we allow ourselves to be fully seen. Not just watched but *witnessed*. To be witnessed is to be acknowledged, and in that acknowledgment, something primal within us awakens. It is a threshold, an unraveling of all the ways we've tried to control how we're perceived.

This was the Dark Feminine rising—the raw, unapologetic hunger to be seen exactly as I was, not softened, not made smaller, not performed into palatability. And it was the Dark Masculine too—the leash, the cage, the steady gaze that refused to look away when I wanted to disappear. These currents collided here. The terror of being too much, and the exquisite truth that being witnessed in that too-muchness was where the power was stirred. There was no role to perform, no script to follow. Just breath, body, and presence. Raw. Unfiltered.

You've probably felt this in your own life. The Dark Feminine, when she's scared of being seen, might cover herself up, make a joke, or try to look "perfect" so no one sees the mess underneath. The Dark Masculine, when distorted, might stare with judgment or pull his attention away to punish. Both leave you feeling smaller.

But when those same instincts are in coherence or unapologetically claimed, the energy shifts completely. The Dark Feminine shows herself as she is—desire, nerves, all of it—and lets it be enough. The Dark Masculine holds steady with his presence, meeting her without turning away.

That's the real edge of visibility. It isn't about whether you like being watched—it's about whether you'll let yourself be fully seen.

I'd never thought of myself as an exhibitionist—in fact, I often judged people who purposely drew attention to themselves—but my body hinted at a different story. The way my nipples tightened against my lingerie, the way my thighs pressed together instinctively, the way my breath hitched at the thought of being unabashedly desired.

To be seen without a filter is to face yourself in a way most people never do. The parts you've softened or reshaped to feel acceptable are stripped away under a gaze that asks for nothing but honesty. And in that honesty, you don't vanish—you take up *more space*. To be fully seen is not just about visibility; it's about recognizing yourself as the raw, unconfined force of who you are.

I *loved* being His prized possession. I loved the way He showed me off, the way He touched me in small, possessive gestures that told the room, *she is mine.*

And still, the voice in my head whispered: This is dangerous.

THE CHILDHOOD ECHOES OF VISIBILITY

I'd been seen before.

On parent-teacher nights, my mother paraded me around like a trophy, basking in the reflected praise from teachers who marveled at my intelligence and obedience. In those moments, I wasn't just a child—I was proof of *her* excellence. I mattered because I made *her* look good.

It had felt good to be noticed, but it had never really been about me.

Even as an adult, when my *More Than Mortal* comic book series took off unexpectedly, my mother asked for copies, only to abandon them unread in a corner of a bookshelf, a token to brag with to her friends. To my knowledge, they still exist there, untouched.

My father was all but absent from my upbringing. I saw him rarely, maybe once a year—no phone calls, no child support. He really had zero active influence on my life except my feeling his absence acutely and believing that I was unwanted by him. On the few occasions I visited him as a child, I always had the feeling that if I became *burdensome,* the visits would cease altogether.

And so I learned: Being seen is conditional. Being valuable means being silent. And *flawless.*

That old programming flickered to life as I leaned in the cage, eyes on me from every direction. Was this any different? Was I simply performing again—this time, for my Dominant instead of my parents?

Or was this something else? I had other childhood experiences that made being the center of attention painful and terrifying. To admit I *liked* this—being seen, being desired—would be to rewrite a fundamental story about myself. It would mean facing the part of me that had spent a lifetime avoiding rejection, horrified of the moment when admiration would turn to exile, because when I had been seen before, it had come at a cost. And yet, here I was. Exposed, owned, and openly lusted after.

A DOOR CRACKING OPEN

This wasn't the moment where everything clicked into place. I didn't walk out of that party declaring myself an exhibitionist. I wasn't ready to claim it yet.

But it was the beginning.

A crack in the foundation of who I thought I was. A question forming in the back of my mind. A door, barely ajar, leading to something I wasn't quite ready to walk through—yet.

To be truly seen is not just about visibility. It's about *sovereignty.* **When you no longer filter yourself through the fear of how you'll be perceived, you step into the highest form of erotic power**. Not a power given or taken, not one performed or proven, but one that simply *is.*

Sovereignty means you don't need to be desired to be powerful. You don't need to be chosen to be worthy. You exist, whole and untamed, whether the world is ready for you or not.

CLOSING THE SCENE: THE MOMENT OF THE FIRST CRACK

Some stories don't shatter in a single moment. They split open slowly—tiny fractures you only notice later, when the light starts seeping through. That night in the cage wasn't a full claiming. But it was a beginning. A fault line running through everything I thought I knew about myself.

I didn't leave with a new identity or a neat label for what I wanted. But I left with a door cracked open, an awareness I couldn't unfeel.

And that's how transformation begins. Not with certainty, but with an opening. An invitation to step closer to the parts of yourself you've been taught to hide.

EROTIC ALCHEMY IN PRACTICE: THE POWER OF BEING SEEN

Embodiment

Stand before a mirror, clothed or unclothed, and hold your own gaze. Notice your breath as you do it. What stories arise—judgments, pride, longing? Stay with them instead of turning away. This is your Dark Feminine asking to be seen, and your Dark Masculine steadying you so you can stay present.

> **Spicy Add-On:** Take one photo of yourself in this state—without editing, without filters, without hiding. Keep it private or share it with someone you trust. The act of being captured adds an erotic edge to being seen.

Integration—Solo

Choose one small way to let yourself be more visible today. Post a photo that feels a little bold, wear clothes that reveal more skin, or share something personal in conversation. Let your Dark Masculine steady the inner tremor: "It's safe to let this be seen."

> **Spicy Add-On:** Take your visibility beyond the private container. Share a piece of yourself in a semi-public way—a bold photo in a safe online group, reading a poem at an open mic, or letting yourself dance with eyes closed at a gathering where others might see. The point isn't shock—it's allowing your Dark Feminine to be witnessed in her hunger and expression, while your Dark Masculine stays stable enough to hold the exposure.

Spicier Add-On: If you want to take it further, self-pleasure in front of a mirror. Let yourself watch. As your arousal rises, whisper what you notice or admire about your body—naming aloud the beauty and power you see.

Integration—Partnered

Invite someone to witness you in a short scene, in person. You might read a piece of writing aloud, dance for them, or undress slowly under their gaze. Their role is not to judge or fix but to simply hold presence. Your role is to let yourself be seen without apology.

Spicy Add-On: Let a trusted partner or friend watch you caress your body or let them choose one item of clothing for you to remove. Play with silence versus words—feel the difference between being watched in complete quiet and being spoken to as they name what they see. See how each changes the charge you experience in your mind and body.

Then, if you're both consenting, switch roles.

CHAPTER 4

PRIMAL UNLEASHED

THE EROTIC POWER OF INSTINCT & ANIMAL DESIRE

I could hear my own breath, sharp and deliberate, as I prowled across the dungeon floor. The atmosphere that night was wilder than usual, almost restless, a current running beneath the black painted walls and the dim lights. Across from me, Justin waited, his body coiled, his eyes locked on me with the same hunger I was pretending not to feel.

We both knew what was coming. The chase. The capture. The inevitable struggle before the surrender.

And then—I would be taken...

THE DAY THE FLOODGATES OPENED

We had negotiated the scene in advance—a capture-and-subdue fantasy that would let me feel the thrill of being hunted, caught, and then claimed. It wasn't about fear, or about dominance in the way most people think of it. It was about the raw *exchange of power* that comes when two equals engage in the most primal of games. The chase was a game.

I felt him coming for me before I saw him. My body lit up before my mind could register.

Adrenaline spiked and I ran—not because I thought I could escape, but because running made what came next inevitable, and that inevitability *turned me on*. Justin was 6'4" and built like a linebacker. There was no question he would win. That was the point.

Primal energy isn't about roles like dominance or submission. It's not about predator and prey or even hunter and hunted. Those labels come later. Primal is older than language, older than culture. It's the body remembering its first language—instinct. The part of you that knows how to move before you think.

When those instincts come up, the Dark currents show through. In distortion, the Dark Feminine might pout, pick a fight, or use her emotions to get her way instead of saying what she really needs. The Dark Masculine, in distortion, might shove past another person's boundaries, talk over them, or use his size and voice to maintain control.

Claimed with care, those same instincts feel very different. The Dark Feminine's hunger becomes simple and clear—asking straight out, reaching for what she wants without apology. The Dark Masculine's drive becomes unshakeable and protective—offering his strength as support, holding ground so others feel safe to let go.

This is the heart of the primal instinct. Left unchecked, it can feel unruly or even hurtful. But when you recognize it and consciously choose it, that same energy shows up as *aliveness*. It's the growl that comes out when someone crosses a line.

The sure grip in your hands when you're holding a child or carrying something heavy for someone else. The raw wanting that spills out of your body when you stop pretending you don't care. These are the places where Dark currents live in all of us.

In its purest form, primal energy dissolves duality. It isn't about choosing between the Dark Feminine's hunger or the Dark Masculine's grip. It's about embodying them together—chaos and structure, wildness and anchor—surging through your body at once, without restraint.

When Justin caught up to me, the impact was hard and deliberate. Delicious. His body closed against mine, pressing me against the wall. My body fought on instinct, thrashing, twisting, my nails catching his arm, my breath ragged. For a flash, I thought I might actually break free. And then his arms closed tighter, pinning me. This wasn't mindless aggression. It was precision. The Dark Masculine in his purest form—weight, presence, command without cruelty. And in me, the Dark Feminine rose to meet him—not as a victim, but as the untamed force that refuses to be small, that growls and writhes and demands: *If you want me, you'd better hold me.*

I fought because it was part of the ritual. Rope. Teeth. Nails. Heat. The sting of skin grabbed, of a slap across my thigh. It was all foreplay.

The Dark Feminine in distortion resists endlessly, afraid to be taken, afraid to *want it*. But in coherence, that resistance is the invitation itself: *Meet me here. Show me you can hold it all.*

It's not just true here. You've probably felt it in your own life, too—pushing back just to see if someone could really hold you.

And Justin did.

I growled, and the reverberation of it sent fire curling through my chest. My breath hitched as he threw me over his shoulder, carried me effortlessly, and then tossed me onto a bed like I weighed nothing at all.

And still, I fought. The struggle before yielding, the illusion of resistance before the body finally lets go. The rope he tied around me was tight but careful, every knot deliberate. *So like him.* His body held me down, his weight an anchor, until I stopped fighting the container and started to feel the joy in it.

His hand slipped between my legs, relentless, insistent. I bucked against him, half-resisting, half needing more.

"Give it over," he growled. "I know you want it."

And he was right. Not just about my body, but about the pleasure I was finally ready to allow. Getting to this place in my life, and in my relationship with him, was a long and hard-won battle. There were years of armoring. Years of believing I had to earn closeness by being useful or impressive. Years of learning how to submit without losing myself—how to be claimed without being erased. Every inch of surrender in that moment was built on the foundation of choosing myself again and again, until I could finally let go on my own terms.

When the orgasm hit, it tore through me. My body convulsed, back arched, sound ripping from my throat as years of control cracked open.

Yes to being taken. Yes to being chosen. Yes to the part of me I had buried under the usefulness and composure.

When the wave subsided, I moved his hand and pulled all of him to me—no resistance left, no hesitation. I opened my legs wide, wanting all of him, claiming my hunger as fiercely as he had claimed me.

Wildness is not just an aesthetic. It's not just an archetype we play at. It's a force of transformation. When I stop trying to *do* primal and simply *become* it, something fundamental shifts. I'm no longer a woman acting out a role. I am the Dark Feminine embodied—raw, unfiltered chaos and hunger. And I am met by the Dark Masculine—the immovable container, the presence that doesn't collapse no matter how much I thrash.

Together, these currents don't cancel each other out. They create the storm.

My surrender wasn't a loss. It was the climax of the game. I had fought just enough to make the moment of yielding feel like the sweetest release. I held the tension on purpose. The more I resisted, the more force I knew the release would carry when I finally let go.

To let myself be untamed isn't recklessness, it's an offering to the part of me that was never meant to be caged, to the energy within me that has always been bigger than the structures designed to contain it. To be untamed is to be in direct communion with the primal pulse of creation itself. The wild doesn't need permission to exist. And neither do I because *I am that*.

You don't need to be in a dungeon to feel this. The Dark Feminine, when she's afraid of her own hunger, might push away what she actually wants, or fight to keep control long past the point where it feels good. The Dark Masculine, in distortion, can let his strength tip into a roughness that overwhelms instead of holds.

But when those same instincts are met with conscious awareness, they carry a different energy. The Dark Feminine's push becomes a test of trust—a way of saying, "Don't just take me when I'm easy, meet me when I'm strong." The Dark Masculine's strength becomes the sturdy pillar that lets the storm happen without anyone getting lost in it.

You've probably felt pieces of this outside of play too—snapping at someone when what you really wanted was closeness or holding space for a friend who needed to rage without falling apart. These are the same dark currents at work. Distortion makes them hurtful. Claimed and coherent, they become the spark that makes connection feel electric and real.

THE WISDOM OF PRIMAL PLAY

Primal play isn't about one person winning and another losing. It's about the charge between the people playing. The moment where power crackles in the air, where both parties know the rules and yet still step into the unknown together.

It is an act of presence. Of raw, unfiltered embodiment. Inside you, there is something wild. And that wildness does not exist in a vacuum. *It thrives in contrast.*

The struggle before giving in. The push before the pull. The moment before the collapse. The hesitation before the leap.

We resist our own pleasure the same way we resist our own primal instincts. We tell ourselves we don't want it, that it's dangerous, that it will cost us something—our dignity, our control, or our carefully crafted self-image.

But when we step into our primal nature, when we *consciously and mindfully* engage in this raw polarity, the animal inside us speaks. We move from decision to instinct, or from hesitation to action. We touch a part of ourselves that is more alive, more knowing, more unfiltered than the self we present to the world.

Instinct isn't just physical; it's energetic. This is where the body becomes a channel, a vessel for something beyond thought. And the more I listen, the more I realize that instinct and intuition are not separate. That what I call *gut feeling* is not just emotional wisdom—it's the language of my energetic body speaking in a way that I was taught to ignore.

This is why primal play is transformative. It is an embodiment of one's fuller expression. When I'm in my primal embodiment, I feel the most in touch with my *yes*—with choice, with hunger and desire, with pleasure—because I'm not filtering any of those things through the eyes of societal expectations or self-judgment.

And the deeper I lean into my primal nature, the more it expands the other aspects of me. It stretches the edges of my duality—where I can be both wild and still.

What if you stopped suppressing your animal nature? What could you unlock if you let yourself move with hunger? To feel, hunt, chase, take, or be taken?

CLOSING THE SCENE: RECLAIMING THE WILD

You were never meant to be fully tamed. Underneath the polished edges and curated self is a body that remembers. A breath that longs to deepen. A growl that has waited lifetimes to be heard.

Your wildness is not something to erase or silence. It's something to court, to seduce you back into your own aliveness.

Because that too-muchness you've tried to control? That's your magic.

So take the leash off your desire. Let your untamed self return home. The wild is not what makes you unsafe.

The suppression of it is.

EROTIC ALCHEMY IN PRACTICE: AWAKENING THE PRIMAL

Embodiment

Stand in front of a mirror and let yourself make sound. Growl, pant, hiss, roar—whatever rises. Notice how your body shifts when your throat is free. Do your shoulders square? Does your chest open? These are your Dark Feminine and Dark Masculine currents waking through raw voice and presence.

> **Spicy Add-On:** Add your hands. Slap your thighs, pull your hair, or drag your nails across your skin while you make sound. Let your body know it's allowed to be wild.

Integration (24-Hour Challenge)

Move as if you were a predator animal. Stalk, crouch, stretch, or prowl across the floor. Then switch—become prey, quick and alert. Notice how your body changes when you shift between roles.

> **Spicy Add-On:** Layer in arousal. Touch yourself like a predator—confident, claiming. Then flip into prey—teasing, tentative, even resisting your own hand before giving in.

Integration—Partnered

Choose someone to explore with. One of you plays predator, the other prey. The predator's role is to chase, pin, or corner; the prey's role is to resist or flee. Keep it playful and safe.

Switch roles if or when you're ready.

Spicy Add-On: When one of you is finally pinned, let it go primal: kissing rough, biting gently, grinding with hunger. The predator holds steady with presence; the prey lets their desire pour out without restraint.

Spicier Add-On: Take it into a more ritual-style hunt. Set a time limit and a defined space (like one room, or the yard at night). The predator prowls, the prey hides or escapes.

When capture happens, the scene moves into agreed erotic territory.

Debrief after to ground back into coherence.

CHAPTER 5

POWER EXCHANGE

HOLDING & BEING HELD

I hadn't planned to tie her. I hadn't planned for any of it. But when she stepped forward—a woman from my kinky pack, *a well-regarded Top and Dominant*—and offered herself to me, something inside me became alert. It was subtle at first, almost quiet. A tingle at my fingertips. A sudden awareness in my breath. The kind of shift that feels small but undeniable, the kind you can't ignore once it's begun.

I had always known myself as submissive. Rope, for me, had meant surrender—being held, being shaped, the paradox of restriction and freedom. But here, standing across from her, a different desire stirred. Not to be tied. To *tie.*

Adrienne looked at me with clear eyes, shoulders relaxed, yet there was something underneath her gaze... a question. A buzz in the space between us. *Will you take me there? Can I surrender into you?*

And suddenly I wanted to say yes. Not with force. Or command. But with presence so full, she could finally stop holding herself up.

The word that came to me was *delicacy.* I didn't want to overpower her. I wanted to hold her so fully that she—this woman who prides herself on holding space for others—forgot the need to hold herself.

This wasn't just about rope. This was about trust.

This was about power.

And surrender.

I stepped off my mat and held my hand out to her.

OOPS, I LIKED IT

I hadn't expected to disappear. But that's exactly what happened.

For months I'd been practicing ropes in workshops and living rooms, memorizing knots, drilling safety checks, rehearsing the mechanics until they felt natural. Rope fascinated me. I loved the contradiction of it—the way it could hold a body firmly and yet invite freedom at the same time. That's what it did for me.

I had never imagined the power it held beyond the physical. I thought that's all it was: skill, structure, practice. I hadn't realized that once rope was on another body, it became something else entirely.

Adrienne stepped onto my mat. We spoke briefly about her body's limitations, her desires and my own. We laughed like friends do, easy and open, but underneath the levity there was weight. She was giving me her trust. She was asking me to lead.

I settled her onto my mat facing away from me. My hands shook slightly as I slipped the blindfold over her eyes. The moment it settled into place, I felt her body exhale, like the first surrender was already happening. I drew her wrists behind her back and looped rope around them. My palms tingled. My chest felt full, like I was holding more than just rope. As I wrapped the first band across her shoulders, she gave me her weight fully. Her spine leaned back into me, her head tilted, and I felt her body whisper: *Yes.*

Something clicked into place. A silent voice rose in me, steady and certain: *I've got you. You can let go.*

The outside world dissolved. My focus narrowed to the rhythm of her breath, the sound of rope sliding across skin, the subtle way her weight shifted as she yielded more deeply. My hands knew what to do, but more than that—my body knew. Every shiver under her skin, every sigh, every pause in her breath was a language I could read.

When she trembled as my breath grazed her neck, I adjusted. When her body pressed back, I tightened. We moved together, her giving, me receiving, me leading, her yielding, until I could no longer tell which one of us had started the dance. The more I invited her to give to me, the more she relaxed. I could almost hear her whisper: *I trust you. I needed this. Thank you.*

This wasn't *practice*. This was ceremony.

Her surrender wasn't a collapse or weakness. It was fierce and deliberate—handing me all of herself because she wanted to, not because she had to. And in me, something new came alive. I didn't feel like I was "in charge." I felt grounded, solid, able to hold everything she gave without flinching.

We weren't playing with rope anymore. We were playing with currents.

I have no idea how long our scene was. Time lost its edge. I tied and untied, tested and held, guided and listened until my hands finally stilled. Finally, I tossed the last coil of rope away and slipped the blindfold from her eyes, cradling her in my arms as we both came back to awareness. She blinked, dazed, soft, open.

Only then did I realize the entire room had gone silent. Dozens of eyes were on us. People who'd been laughing, playing, and wrestling had all stopped. They were staring, breathless, drawn into the rhythm that had carried us.

Her surrender was so total that the whole room could feel it. My steadiness was so anchored that everyone around us picked up on it, even if they couldn't explain why.

We all let out a collective breath.

My cheeks flushed hot under the weight of their gaze, but it wasn't shame. It was awe.

For the first time in my life, I understood what real power was.

THE TRUTH ABOUT POWER EXCHANGE

Most people think power exchange is about control. About who commands and who obeys, or who takes and who gives.

But the truth is, those are just costumes. What's underneath is far more profound.

Power exchange is not simply about dominance and submission. It is archetypal. The unconscious Domme/Dominant may seek control to soothe their fear. The unconscious submissive may yield out of unworthiness. But the Dark Feminine doesn't surrender from weakness—she chooses to dissolve into the One who can meet her, the One who won't collapse under her intensity. And the Dark Masculine doesn't lead so he can overpower—he leads to elevate, to create the container that makes such surrender possible. This is the real game. Not a hierarchy of roles, but an alchemy of currents.

True power exchange isn't force. It's presence. It's the ability to read the body in front of you, to feel the unspoken signals, to guide someone deeper into themselves without pushing them past their capacity.

In that rope scene, I wasn't dictating or commanding. I was listening with every cell of my body, anticipating before she moved, adjusting before she asked.

This is attunement. This is power exchange.

Not force, not control. Presence.

Whether in dominance and submission, primal play, rope, or even everyday relationships, **power exchange is an act of energetic leadership.**

This is what I refer to as D/S—with a capital "S." Submission as a state, or as a frequency. Power exchange, engaged in this way, is ceremony. A conscious offering of one God to Another. D/S is about choosing, with full agency, to play at the edge of power and devotion together.

Up until then, I had only understood service from inside submission—what it meant to give myself over, or to surrender. But in this moment, standing as the one She trusted to take the lead, I realized service could be sacred from the other side too. To Top in this way wasn't about control—it was about receiving Her trust as an offering, and honoring it with precision and reverent presence. The "S" was also *service*, but I was beginning to understand its fullness: that both offering trust and holding it with integrity were sacred acts.

Power exchange doesn't just exist in kink, either. It exists in every aspect of life. Whether in a boardroom, in a dance, or in a whispered *yes* between lovers, power is always being exchanged. The question is—are you aware of it?

And whether you identify as a Dominant, a submissive, a switch, or simply as someone navigating the intricacies of human connection, the same principle applies: True power is not in the holding. True surrender is not in the losing. **The magic is in the meeting.**

THE MIND IS THE FIRST ROPE: THE POWER OF THE MINDFUCK

Rope, as powerful as it is, isn't even necessary. Some of the most intense exchanges of power happen without a single knot.

A whispered order. The snap of a belt in the dark. The denial of an orgasm stretched to the point of madness. These things tie up the mind more powerfully than any rope.

Because real surrender isn't just physical, it's mental. It's the moment you stop tracking time, stop anticipating outcomes, stop holding yourself up, and simply let yourself be carried. The *mindfuck* is the art of making someone question what they know, what they expect, and what they believe will happen next.

When you give over control, you're not just giving your body—you're giving your trust. The mindfuck amplifies this by making you question how and when the next moment will arrive.

ENERGY EXCHANGE VERSUS POWER EXCHANGE

Many confuse *energy exchange* with *power exchange,* but they're not the same. Energy exchange is the interplay of sensation and emotion and awareness between people. It happens in every interaction—whether platonic, romantic, or erotic. It's the current of electricity in a shared glance or the charge felt in deep conversation.

Power exchange, on the other hand, involves a deliberate dynamic of clear power roles—one leads and one yields. Unlike energy exchange, which is fluid and unstructured, power exchange follows an agreed-upon framework where one person holds space in a way that allows the other to let go.

When I tied Adrienne, the energy between us was undeniable. Every sigh, every shift of weight, every tremor under the rope was energy moving through both of us. That's energy exchange. But what made that scene different—the reason the room went silent—was power exchange. It wasn't just the energy moving. It was *direction*. It was current flowing through the container. I wasn't just receiving her energy; I was shaping it, guiding it, holding it so she could go deeper. She wasn't just feeling me; she was offering her power into my hands, knowing I could hold it.

Both are powerful. Both are transformative. But power exchange has an added element of intentionality—of *choosing to create a container where surrender can deepen.*

Energy exchange is everywhere. A glance across the room. A heated conversation. A kiss. But power exchange requires conscious choice. One leads. One yields. Both step in willingly, and with that agreement, something bigger than either of them takes over. To yield deeply requires immense strength. To hold power with integrity requires immense responsibility.

This is the first threshold of erotic medicine—the willingness to dissolve so that something new may emerge.

POWER EXCHANGE AS A PATH TO TRANSCENDENCE

People think transcendence comes from hours of meditation, chanting, fasting, or ritual. And yes, those things work. But transcendence can also come from rope.

Because I was tying her, I lost myself. My mind dissolved into sensation, into rhythm, into the sound of her breath. There was no clock, no room, no thought about who was watching. There was only presence.

That's the path mystics describe—the surrender of mind to body, of ego to union.

Power exchange allows us to touch the Mystery. It is a spiritual act disguised as an erotic one. At that moment, I wasn't tying rope. I was being tied to the Mystery itself. She wasn't surrendering to me. She was surrendering *through* me. This is the truth of power exchange. Not a hierarchy, but a dance. A meeting of two forces that together create something neither could access alone.

This is why I insist that power exchange isn't about roles or dynamics. The Dark Feminine doesn't yield because she's small. She yields because she knows that in the right container, she can become infinite. The Dark Masculine doesn't lead to control. He leads because steadiness opens the door for both of them to know God.

CLOSING THE SCENE: POWER AS AN ACT OF PRESENCE

We're taught that yielding means weakness, and control means strength. Power exchange—whether through rope, touch, words, or another form of leadership—reveals the opposite.

It's not about force or about who wins. It is about meeting someone exactly where they are and holding them there without forcing them forward or pulling them back. It's about trusting yourself to lead without ego and to follow without fear.

When we understand this, we stop *playing* at power and we start *embodying* it.

Presence says: I see you. I can hold you. You can let go.

EROTIC ALCHEMY IN PRACTICE: HOLDING & BEING HELD

Embodiment

Stand tall and place one hand *firmly* on your chest, the other *lightly* on your belly. Feel the difference in weight and pressure. The hand on your chest represents the Dark Masculine—strong, structured, protective. The hand on your belly represents the Dark Feminine—sensitive, expressive, alive.

Shift pressure between the two and notice the contrast—how firm touch feels different from light touch, how each changes your breath or body awareness. Let the difference itself become the conversation between these two currents.

> **Spicy Add-On:** Take this into self-pleasure. Use one hand with firm, steady pressure—stroking, squeezing, or holding in a way that feels like the Dark Masculine's containment. With the other, bring a lighter, teasing touch—circling, brushing, gliding like the Dark Feminine's playfulness.
>
> Let your body feel the contrast, then weave them together—pressure and play, structure and flow. Notice how arousal shifts when both currents meet.

Integration—Solo

Choose one place in your daily life where you usually hold back—maybe speaking up in a meeting, asking for support, or showing affection. Let your Dark Feminine lead: Say the thing, make the ask, express what you usually swallow. Then pause and invite your Dark Masculine to meet her: Notice how your feet ground, how your tone clarifies, how your body steadies as you stand in your truth.

> **Spicy Add-On:** Close the door, put on music that stirs you, and let your Dark Feminine erupt. Speak the desires or confessions you usually censor. Let your hips grind, your voice rise, your hands clutch at air or skin.
>
> When the energy crests, let your Dark Masculine cut through—plant your feet, grip a chair or wall, and drop one word or phrase like a lightning strike: *"Enough." "Here." "Mine."* Feel how the two currents ignite each other inside you.

Integration—Partnered

Invite someone you trust into a scene. Take turns leading and following. The one leading embodies the Dark Masculine—steady eye contact, grounded stance, clear words: "I've got you." "Keep going." The one being held embodies the Dark Feminine: letting their voice, their body, or their truth move more fully than usual.

Then switch. Notice how the energy of power and devotion shifts between you.

> **Spicy Add-On:** Stand facing each other and let your bodies "argue" without words. Keep it physical and simple: One presses in with their chest or shoulder, the other either yields, pivots, or pushes back. Trade off initiating. Stay primal—press, lean, grab, yield—without overthinking.

After a few rounds, pause and notice the energy underneath. The Dark Feminine often shows up in the push, pull, and provocation. The Dark Masculine often shows up in the grounding, holding, and containing. Switch initiators again and feel how quickly this can shift from playful roughhousing into erotic charge.

PART TWO: TRANSMUTATION

THE EDGE OF PLEASURE & PAIN

CHAPTER 6

THE ART OF RESTRAINT

ROPE, STILLNESS, AND DEEP SURRENDER

The first knot is just a whisper, a suggestion against the skin. The second carries weight, pulling you deeper. By the third, the rope has made its claim. The more it gathers you in, the clearer it becomes. This is no half-measure: You're not going anywhere.

At first, panic might flare, a quickening of breath, a rush of heat in the chest. But almost as quickly, something else rises. Relief. Release. A deep exhale that seems to come from the bones. Because, for once, you don't have to move. You don't have to decide. You don't have to hold everything together.

Someone else is holding it all for you.

Restraint is not just about restriction—like power exchange, it's about trust. The kind of trust that lets you stop guarding against imagined threats. The kind of trust that makes your body soften in a way you didn't know it needed.

Like the blindfold restricting sight, when you can't move, you can let go.

HOW DO YOU WANT TO FEEL?

I bottomed for a friend in rope practice one day. Nothing formal—just a typical rope lab, the kind I went to two or three times a week. This was the first time David had tied me, and while I knew he was still learning, I trusted him.

As always, we went through negotiation: injuries, flexibility, boundaries, the usual technical checklist. My body relaxed, ready for the familiar rhythm of rope. But then he asked me something no one had ever asked before:

"How do you want to feel by the end of this scene?"

I blinked at him, caught off guard.

Rope had always been a place of safety to me—the same kind of safety I felt with a blindfold, where I could disappear, held in the comfort of compression, wrapped in the quiet stillness of being bound. It was like swaddling—a return to innocence, and deeply soothing.

Normally, I might have said I wanted to feel sexy or desired. Or perhaps powerful. But in that moment, with him watching me carefully, something broke through the surface.

"I want to feel cared for."

I felt my throat tighten as I said it, a flicker of shame mixed with relief. To ask for care—especially in a space so often charged with dominance, power, and sex—felt almost rebellious.

But he didn't blink. He nodded. Quiet, steady, sure.

He abandoned any kind of dominance or erotic charge and stepped into something even more intimate: pure attention. Presence. He tied with quiet determination, his hands sure, his breath calm. The rope slid across my skin, scratchy at first, then warming with the heat of my body. Each wrap was deliberate, not rushed, not careless.

As the rope crossed my chest, pulled tight around my arms, I felt my shoulders drop. My breath slowed. The tension I didn't even know I was carrying began to dissolve.

I could feel my own emotions swell at the simplicity of it: the feeling of being supported. Safe.

Every shift in me, he met. Every sigh, every twitch, he felt and adjusted to. He didn't flinch or turn away. His presence steadied me the way a strong tree steadies the earth around it.

This rope wasn't about control. It wasn't about restriction. It was about *holding*—not in a limiting way, but in the way a strong foundation holds a house, or in the way a riverbank holds a river, allowing it to flow deeper, stronger.

In me, the Dark Feminine showed up as the part that just wanted to stop holding it all together, to relax and be cared for without shame. In him, the Dark Masculine showed up as a steady presence—not flinching and not looking away, just holding me exactly as I was.

I realized then that this was the true power of restraint: the simple comfort of being held, and the sacred experience of being fully and deeply attended to.

WHY WE CRAVE RESTRAINT

Bondage is one of the most universal kinks, appearing everywhere—from silk scarves tied around wrists to elaborate rope suspensions. But its power goes far beyond the physical because restraint is another paradox.

To be held in place is to feel a unique kind of freedom. When movement is no longer yours to control, you drop into yourself in a way that's rarely possible otherwise.

It forces stillness. In a world that demands constant movement, being tied, cuffed, or made to hold still invites a kind of surrender we don't often allow ourselves. Stillness magnifies awareness. It strips away the need to act or to respond—and replaces it with pure being.

Allowing yourself to be restrained can deepen trust. There's a profound intimacy in letting someone else hold your body still, in letting yourself rest inside their strength. The Dark Feminine, so often judged for her chaos and hunger, can finally relax into the Dark Masculine's unwavering presence—because she knows she won't be dropped.

Restraint shifts your experience of pleasure. When you can't move, touch feels different. Every bind tightening, every pause, every breath against your neck becomes amplified. It forces you into a deep, embodied presence.

Bondage also creates a ritual of release. When your body is held, your mind follows. It's no longer about what comes next—it is about what *is*. This is why so many people experience catharsis in rope. It's softening. A *breaking open*.

ROPE AS RITUAL: THE ART OF BEING HELD

Some forms of bondage focus on control. But at its highest expression—rope is something else entirely.

Rope is meditation. The rhythm of knots, the slow slide of fiber across skin, the ever-increasing tension—it creates a trance state. An altered way of being.

It's also an art form. It's sculpture with bodies, a silent conversation, a form of deep listening. A conscious, skilled rigger is not just someone who ties well. They're someone who can hear a shift in breath, feel a change in muscle, sense when the body wants to give more.

When the Dark Feminine thrashes, the rigger doesn't fight against her—they simply hold. When she softens, they soften too. The Dark Masculine here isn't rigid authority—it's steady responsiveness.

And in that meeting, rope becomes a ritual.

BEYOND ROPE: THE MANY FORMS OF RESTRAINT

Restraint doesn't always mean rope. There are many ways to play with restriction, each with its own energy and impact.

- Handcuffs & Metal Restraints—The cold bite of steel against skin, the decisive click of a lock—metal restraints bring immediacy, a shift in power you can hear.
- Body Weight & Physical Pinning—Sometimes restraint isn't about equipment. Sometimes it's nothing more than a body pressing down on another, wrists pinned above a person's head. Primal. Inescapable. A surge of Dark Feminine fight meeting the Dark Masculine's unceasing hold.
- Scarves, Belts, & Everyday Objects—A scarf looped around wrists, a belt cinched snugly across the

waist—these forms of restraint bring sensuality into the mix, transforming the everyday into the erotic.

- Sensory Deprivation & Restraint—A blindfold paired with tied wrists, or noise-canceling headphones combined with cuffs—each layer strips away another form of control, amplifying what remains.
- Suspension & Extreme Bondage—Being lifted off the ground, your weight carried by rope, offers the ultimate paradox: bound yet weightless, held yet free. A complete surrender to gravity, the rigger, and the void itself.

CLOSING THE SCENE: THE PARADOX OF RESTRAINT

To be held is to be free.

Restraint is not just about surrendering movement—it's about surrendering to *trust*.

When you cannot move, you have no choice but to feel. And in that stillness, in that deep presence, you stop *doing* and start *being*.

The Dark Feminine, when she doesn't have to hold herself up anymore, can finally take a breath. The Dark Masculine, when he holds without collapsing, gives her that space. Together they show the paradox of restraint: the tighter the binding, the deeper the freedom.

EROTIC ALCHEMY IN PRACTICE: TRUSTING THE BIND

Embodiment

Let yourself be restrained in a simple, safe way—a scarf looped around your wrists, a blanket tucked snugly over you, or a partner using their body weight to hold you still. Notice what happens when movement is gone. Do your muscles fight? Does your breath catch? Or does something soften?

> **Spicy Add-On:** Once restrained, let the one holding you hover and tease—hands close but not landing, lips brushing without kissing, fingers tracing only to pull away. The denial sharpens stillness and turns surrender into ache.

Integration—Solo (24-Hour Challenge)

For one day, practice "restraint" in ordinary life. When the impulse to grab your phone, interrupt your flow, or reach for a snack arises, pause. Place your hands in your lap, take three slow breaths, and let the urge rise and fall without acting on it. Notice how your body shifts when you hold yourself instead of giving in right away.

> **Spicy Add-On:** If you're playing with self-pleasure, keep your toy or your hands hovering, just out of reach, every time the urge spikes. Breathe through the ache for a few minutes before giving in. Notice how restraint makes the eventual touch sharper, hotter, and more consuming.

Integration—Partnered

Invite someone into a restraint scene. One person holds the other—one pinning the other gently, tucking them under a blanket, or keeping their wrists loosely bound. The one restrained practices surrendering their weight, trusting the other to track breath, tension, and comfort. The one holding practices the Dark Masculine current—leading, adjusting pressure, and noticing what it feels like to hold responsibility for another's body.

When you're done, switch roles if you choose.

> **Spicy Add-On:** Layer in arousal. The one holding chooses when—or if—the restrained one receives touch: stroking, kissing, stimulating at their own pace. Play with denial or edging: Pause before any pleasure peaks, or just stretch the arousal out longer than the restrained one would choose for themselves.

CHAPTER 7

POLARITY PLAY

THE ALCHEMY OF OPPOSITES

We often seek transformation through external rituals, altered mind-states, or deep spiritual practice—but the most profound initiations happen *in the body*. Through polarity play, we enter a space where the self dissolves, where instinct overrides thought, and where we touch something far more ancient than identity.

We think of power as something fixed—held or surrendered, possessed or given away. But true power isn't static. It's a dance, a doorway—a dynamic current shaped by energy and intent.

A BIRTHDAY IN HIGH PROTOCOL

It was my birthday, but the gift was not mine to receive. It was mine to *give*.

At the time, I had a husband, Matt—and I also had a Dominant. The three of us had crafted this dynamic carefully, with intention and love. My husband and I had discovered that true D/s would never work between us. Too much history, and too many threads of partnership and codependency.

But my Dominant… He existed in a different space in my life. When we were together, I could step into something else entirely: submission that felt uncompromised.

It was still early in our dynamic. My husband was away on a business trip that week, so for my birthday, my Dominant suggested a full day of *high protocol.*

I had heard the term before, but at the time it was just a nebulous concept of structure and discipline.

Two days before, He sent me a list of instructions. A meal to prepare. A cocktail to perfect. And then a few small, strange requests: that I brush my teeth with the opposite hand, and that I tie my shoes in reverse order. At first, they seemed silly, almost arbitrary. But as the day unfolded, I discovered the depth beneath them.

Each request disrupted habit. Each one forced awareness. Brushing my teeth clumsily with my left hand slowed me down. Tying my shoes backward snapped me out of autopilot. What seemed insignificant became a spell—shifting my attention, reminding me He was with me in every movement.

By the time I walked through the grocery store for ingredients, I realized I'd thought of Him with every step. He was there in the produce aisle, in the clink of glassware I chose for His drink, in the rhythm of my body as I moved through the day.

The anticipation wrapped around me like invisible rope.

I prepared the space. Sent pictures documenting each step—the fresh ingredients I'd selected, the clothing I chose, the setting of the outdoor table.

When He arrived, my focus was singular: Serve.

He led me outside to the pool deck and instructed me to kneel. The concrete was warm from the sun but rough against my knees, so He had me lay a towel down for cushion. It wasn't exactly comfortable—especially not in the heels I wore. My thighs trembled and my toes clenched against the soles of my shoes, but the discomfort became its own kind of fun, an edge I leaned into as I learned more about myself in this role.

I knelt at His feet, waiting. The aches in my knees sharpened my presence.

Serve from the left.
Refill from the right.
Move slowly, deliberately.
Don't anticipate—wait.

Within the formality, something opened. The relief of being fully present. Watchful but not anticipating. The formality gave me structure I could rest in, each instruction a frame that quieted my mind. His focused attention anchored me, reminding me that I mattered. And in that paradox I felt the truth: that in serving Him, I was also serving myself. Every act felt whole on its own—pouring, waiting, kneeling—made meaningful and complete by His attention and my surrender.

And then, as if to deepen that rhythm of service, He offered to teach me how to clean and shine His leather dress shoes. He spoke with the calm authority of a man who had done this a hundred times before—lessons carried from His years in the Navy. How to set the polish just right. How to use the cloth in small, steady circles. How patience and pressure created the shine. Each instruction was precise, methodical, and carried the weight of ritual.

Something new bloomed inside my chest. I'd always been fascinated by *erotic bootblacking*—the deeply sensual, almost meditative act of caring for leather that bordered on worship. But this was more than skill-building. This was His time, His undivided attention… His true birthday offering to me.

As I knelt there polishing leather, a space in me filled that I hadn't known was empty. A space left behind by an absent father and an overworked mother. By childhood wounds of incest, neglect, and emotional and verbal abuse. I wasn't feeling like a child at this moment, but I was feeling noticed and cherished, guided in a way that healed something very old, or perhaps *young*, inside of me.

And beneath it all, the currents stirred.

He'd stepped into the Dark Masculine—sturdy, precise, creating the container I could relax inside. And I'd stepped into the Dark Feminine—still, open, letting myself be received instead of performing or demanding.

The structure didn't confine me. It freed me.

Ritual didn't just amplify the erotic—it awakened the archetypal. And there was a delicious reverence in that.

THE SACRED TECHNOLOGY OF RITUAL & PROTOCOL

Ritual and protocol often dance together in D/s, but they are not the same.

Protocol is structure. It's the Dark Masculine at work—the form that says: *Here is the container. Here is the frame. This is where your energy can move, and I will not let it fall apart.* Protocol is repeatable, predictable, and concrete. It gives the outline of what will happen: how you kneel, what words you say, which gestures mark the beginning and end.

Ritual is the spark inside that form. It's the Dark Feminine charge—the breath of meaning that animates the structure. Ritual turns protocol from mechanics into magic. It's what transforms kneeling into devotion, posture into prayer, or gesture into offering.

Think of protocol as the stage directions; ritual is the emotion and presence that make the play alive. Protocol says *do this in this way*. Ritual says *this is what it means*.

On my birthday, everything was drenched in ritual. Protocol created the stage. Ritual made it sacred.

In those moments, I wasn't just serving or obeying Him. I was *reverencing Him.* And that reverence was being consciously *received by Him, and then reflected back to me.*

This isn't confined to D/s. I've had protocols with romantic partners that weren't part of any formal power exchange. One lover always opened my car door, snapped my seatbelt into place, and then opened the door again when it was time to exit the car. Before I got in or stepped out, we'd pause—look each other in the eyes—and share a kiss.

It wasn't about obedience or control. It was about honoring each other. Every time we did it, we were consciously acknowledging our bond. Sometimes we got lazy. One of us would skip the moment. But with just a longer gaze or a deeper kiss, we'd bring each other back. Back to presence. Back to the meaning underneath the act.

That's what protocol can do. It holds a space for remembrance. It says: *This isn't just habit. This is intention.*

Protocol can also exist in non-romantic or community settings. A person taking their hat off at the dinner table, friends who share a secret handshake, healers who open and close a session with words or a gesture—all are engaging this technology. Even in spiritual traditions—bowing before an altar, smudging the body, or placing objects in a specific order—we're using protocol and ritual to create coherence.

When done with devotion, protocol becomes a bridge to something bigger. It says, Here is the container. Enter it with presence and let intention and ritual make it sacred.

This is how we make the taboo sacred again.

THE ART OF EROTIC SERVICE

Not all who love to serve are submissive, just like not all who love to lead are Dominants.

Service is an orientation, not a role. It's a way of saying: *This moment matters. You matter. Let me show you.* This is one of the most misunderstood distinctions in erotic and relational dynamics, especially in kink. People often conflate the desire to be of service with the desire to submit. But they are not the same.

I've met individuals—feminine, masculine, queer, straight, and everything in between—who come alive in acts of service. I've felt it in erotic bootblacking, in the slow glide of a cloth across leather. But I've also felt it in a lover who lit scented candles and ran me a bath after a long day. In a friend who quietly folded my laundry when I was too raw to function.

Service becomes sacred when it is intentional.

The Dark Feminine shines here—her devotion, her presence, her full-bodied offering of self. The Dark Masculine receives with steadfastness, honoring her offering as a gift rather than diminishment. And sometimes, the polarity flips: The Masculine serves through structure and leadership, while the Feminine receives and acknowledges that leadership.

Either way, the current of service is holy.

Erotic bootblacking is just one expression. But so is offering a glass of water with both hands. So is kneeling to slip off someone's shoes after a long night. So is the deliberate, wordless choice to *pour yourself into another person's pleasure,* not because you're less than, but because you are already full.

MORE THAN AN OBJECT: THE TABOO OF OBJECTIFICATION

Objectification is one of the most misunderstood kinks because it can look like dehumanization. But when it is chosen, it is an extreme form of surrender and offering.

To be objectified is to become a vessel, to give yourself over as art, furniture, or possession—not because you want to be diminished, but because you want to be magnified. To exist entirely for Someone Else's pleasure is to feel yourself seen, prized, and cherished in a way that dissolves shame. The taboo turns to medicine: the very act of being claimed fills the hunger to belong, to matter, or to be made into something worthy of display.

I have experienced this in subtle ways—kneeling at a Dominant's feet or held in stillness as Their possession and existing only for Their pleasure. But I've also seen people turned into a living dinner table, a piece of art, or a body shown off as a statement of ownership—like that night my Dominant put me on display in that cage.

The Dark Feminine comes alive here—not smaller, but braver, daring to show herself without a filter. The Dark Masculine meets her by staying, not looking away, and treating that moment as worthy of reverence.

FROM SUBMISSION TO HOLDING POWER: THE AWAKENING OF BOTHNESS

For years, submission was my home. It gave me presence, devotion, the sacred gift of surrender. But the deeper I went, the more something unexpected stirred—a hunger to *hold power* as fully as I had once surrendered to it.

At first, I resisted. It wasn't a rejection of my submission, nor a desire to abandon it. It was about wholeness.

Submission had taught me how to listen. How to stay with sensation instead of fleeing. How to quiet my breath and meet intensity without collapsing. And those same skills were exactly what power required.

True power wasn't control. True surrender wasn't weakness. Both were courage, both were presence, both were divine.

STEPPING INTO AUTHORITY: A DAY IN POWER

The first time someone knelt for me and asked me to take control, I hesitated. Another member of my kinky pack was struggling. She carried a weight of some unspoken anxiety, a tension she couldn't shake, and she came to me with a request: Would I put her in submission for a day?

She was a petite but powerful woman—a martial artist, fierce and independent.

I collared her with her own collar—a symbol of structure and safety for her. She softened immediately. And from that moment on, she and the day belonged to Me.

I had her draw Me a bath, wash Me, dry Me, and help Me dress. I saw how she softened, how the tension melted from her body as she settled into the container I built.

I took her to a fine dining restaurant and ordered *for us*. When the food arrived at the table, I had her prepare our plates—she waited for Me to begin eating before starting herself. Paying attention to these protocols kept her out of her head. I made decisions for her, removing the weight of choice so she could rest fully in her surrender.

When we returned home, we moved into restraint and sensation play. I bound her, feeling the power shift more deeply as she surrendered to My rope, My hands, My flogger, My crop... My *authority*. No fear—only relief.

I moved her to a hard point, clipped her to the stainless steel ring that hung from the ceiling, and applied a vibrator to the swollen bits over her panties.

At first, she leaned into the restraint and the pleasure. We both did. I loved forced orgasm—both giving and receiving—and watching people climax. But eventually, the sensation built and became overwhelming for her. She started to struggle against me.

I have a touch of sadist in me, especially when it comes to overdelivering sensation. I used my body weight to keep her from escaping as I directed the toy even more intensely against her most sensitive parts.

Her Dark Feminine chaos surged, hungry, untamed. She strained harder. My Dark Masculine held steady, unflinching, present. I held her gaze. Watched her face register my unspoken message: *I've got you. Surrender.*

She fought for a few more tense moments and then, finally, she let go. I saw the shift the instant it happened—her shoulders slumping, her body sagging heavier into the restraints, no longer holding herself up but letting them hold her for me. The resistance drained away as she gave herself over—to the sensations crashing through her, to her own desire, and to Me. I watched the sudden overload of neurotransmitters and sensations move through her mind and body. She unraveled, eyes rolling into the back of her head, her head lolling backward.

I held her through every wave of intensity and release until I decided she was done. And that's when I felt something profound settle in Me, because I knew:

I was capable of *both*. Of dissolving and of containing.

Polarity was never about choosing one side—it was about the reach itself. The dance between opposites, each straining toward the other, pulling us closer to completion. To play at the edge of polarity is to feel the hunger for wholeness. And when those currents meet—one dissolving, one holding steady—the opening is not just between two people. It is a doorway into the divine.

CLOSING THE SCENE: THE ALCHEMY OF OPPOSITES

Polarity play isn't about hierarchy. It's about meeting.

The Dark Feminine doesn't submit because she's weak. She submits because her hunger wants to be met. The Dark Masculine doesn't lead to control. He leads because his containment gives her wildness something to push against. Together they don't cancel each other out—they spark.

Power and surrender are mirrors rather than opposites. Polarity creates the invitation to become whole.

EROTIC ALCHEMY IN PRACTICE: THE DANCE OF GIVING & RECEIVING

Embodiment

Choose one simple ritual act—pouring tea, setting a plate, opening a door. Slow it down. Notice how posture, eye contact, intention, and breath change the meaning of the act. Feel what happens when you let this ordinary gesture carry a tone of devotion.

> **Spicy Add-On:** Write out a short erotic service scene. Imagine one character serving—kneeling, pouring a drink, undressing, or presenting something like an offering—and the other receiving. Let the words be simple and sensory. It doesn't need to be a full story—just a sketch that makes you feel the heat of service—from either side—in your body.

Integration—Solo

Create an ongoing micro-protocol for yourself. It could be lighting incense before journaling, pausing with a hand on your stomach before meals, or setting your glass down with care after every sip. Treat this repeated act as an anchor into presence.

> **Spicy Add-On**: Create a secret ritual around self-pleasure. It might be always lighting the same candle, using the same pillow, or taking the same kneeling posture before touching yourself. Treat it as worship: of your body, of your desire, or of your own erotic sovereignty.

Integration—Partnered

Offer someone a service—pouring their drink, removing their shoes, preparing something they enjoy. Do it deliberately, without rush or expectation. Let them simply receive.

Then trade, letting them serve you while you practice staying open and receptive.

> **Spicy Add-On:** Offer a sensual service: slowly undressing another person, feeding them a bite of fruit, or kneeling to present a drink. Keep it precise, attentive, almost ceremonial. The eroticism comes not from what you do, but from the reverence you bring to doing it.
>
> Then switch.

CHAPTER 8

EROTIC SHADOWS

RECLAIMING THE MONSTER

In kink, we often talk about the shame of masochism—the fear of being broken, of being too much, of wanting pain at all. But there's another shame that cuts just as deep and is spoken of far less.

The shame of wanting to hurt. The shame of wanting to *take*.

Masochists are often granted sympathy—their desires can be framed as catharsis or purification. But sadists? Sadists are feared or distrusted, even vilified.

THE SHAME OF WANTING TO HURT

What kind of person enjoys causing pain?

For many, that question festers. It makes them wonder if something is broken inside of them. It makes them afraid of their own hands, their own hunger, and their own pleasure. And worst of all, it makes them afraid to share themselves fully with the people they trust.

I never carried as much shame about my sadism as I did about my masochism or my sexual desire, and I think that's because I was exposed to people with darker sadistic appetites than my own—and because I was grateful for the role these sadists played for the masochist in me. I've known people who craved giving pain in ways that made my sadist feel delicate by comparison. And that larger perspective—the understanding that sadistic desire lives on such a vast spectrum—allowed me to judge myself less.

But I've also known many who struggled with self-judgment.

I knew a sadist who needed aftercare after a scene as much as their bottom did, if not *more*. Not because they regretted the play, but because they needed time to re-acclimate. To shift from *beast mode* back to *baseline humanity*. And to be reminded that they were not a monster.

And that, I think, is what so many sadists fear: that their unique brand of pleasure makes them something to be feared. That if they let go fully, they will lose themselves.

But what if the real danger isn't in feeling too much, but in suppressing too much? When we deny or repress our darker desires, they don't disappear—they fester, emerging in ways we don't, or sometimes *can't*, control. But *conscious, intentional play*—meeting the edge with care—teaches us how to calibrate sensation, to know exactly what the line is. To own our hunger without shame.

Because shame thrives in secrecy. And secrecy is what makes desire reckless.

THE BREAKING—A MASOCHIST'S RELEASE

I remember the night I broke.

My pack and I—hungry, dirty wolves—had been playing together for months—learning each other's bodies, exploring each other's edges. Nearly three nights a week, we practiced—*biting, flogging, spanking, tying*. Tested each other. Built our tolerance, pushed our limits, fucked up, tried again...

That night, it was my turn. Rob—a steady, skilled Top—stood behind me. The rest of the pack formed a loose circle, not intervening, just watching, holding energy like witnesses at a ritual fire.

My body had learned to give and hold pain like an accolade, a trophy of my own badassery. I found value in being a warrior, in *enduring* and proving that I could hold everything that was given to me.

He struck. Slowly at first. Then harder. Fists, implements, open hand...

Pain has a rhythm, and He played it like music—building in waves, easing, then crashing down again. I wanted to be a gladiator. I wanted to leave the scene victorious, body marked, chest high. I thought strength meant withstanding. Enduring. Outlasting. I could feel my body responding, my nervous system adjusting, riding the endorphin drop only to rise again.

He pushed me. Took me to edge after edge. When He reached the peak of what He thought I could take, He'd push me just a little higher. I had techniques I'd developed for exactly this, but even those were being stretched.

But then He took me past what I thought I could hold. A strike that buckled me and stole my breath. I wasn't a gladiator anymore. I was a trembling animal, broken open.

My body gave out before my mind could cling to control. I collapsed—

Not onto the ground—His arms were there first. He caught me before my knees hit. I shook and sobbed in His embrace, guttural sounds tearing out of me, decades of grief and rage I didn't know I was carrying.

I cried and cried. For the next hour, my pack passed me around like something sacred, cradling me in their arms. *Holding me but never asking anything of me.* They didn't ask me to explain. They didn't try to fix it. They simply held me until I was emptied.

I wish I could say I always let myself be seen this honestly. But the truth is, I often prided myself on being the one who could take it all, even when I was cracking inside. That was my own Dark Feminine shadow—hiding the depth of my need beneath the mask of the unbreakable masochist.

I hadn't known how much I had been carrying until I was drained of it. And when the sobs finally stopped that night, I felt… weightless.

That break wasn't about pain. It was about release. It was the moment my masochism shifted from being a performance of strength into a portal of feeling.

What I didn't realize then was how directly it traced back to childhood. To losing my brother at fifteen. To the incest memories of him that surfaced that same year. To my decision to protect my mother by silencing myself, freezing my rage and grief so she wouldn't fall apart. I shut my own body down to survive. Pain became my way back to life.

Masochism cracked that shell wide open. Each intense sensation, each sharp sting, became a way to reconnect with myself, to reclaim the body that had become foreign, unfeeling territory. It helped break through decades of emotional armor. When Rob finally "broke me," it wasn't about the physical release—it was about decades of trapped emotion and ancestral and past-life trauma, all finally granted permission to rise and *move through me.*

That night, the Dark Feminine rose in me—as the force that breaks masks, rips open what was buried, and births the truth. And the Dark Masculine was there too—not only in Rob's steady arms catching me as I fell apart, but in the circle of my pack. One by one, they held me, anchored me, passed me gently around like a sacred object. Their presence became the structure, the container that would not let me shatter. Together, they embodied the unshakable current that steadied my storm.

For so long, I thought my value lived in how much I could take. I wore endurance like a crown, proof of my worthiness. But the truth is, that was just my ego performing toughness, afraid to admit how much I needed to actually fall apart.

WHEN MY SADIST STEPPED FORWARD

Another night. Another scene.

Casey wanted me to hurt her. To push her to that blurred line where pain and pleasure become indistinguishable. To draw something out of her she couldn't reach alone.

I knew that hunger.

I cuffed her. Restrained her to the cross. My hands, claws, a paddle, my whip.

She struggled. Moaned. Begged for more. Face slaps.

Hair pulling. More impact play.

Then I did something new. Something new for me.

I grabbed her chin, forced her eyes to mine, and whispered: "I want you to count down from ten. Slowly. Everything we just did? That was for you. These last ten… they're for Me."

Her body shuddered. I watched her take a breath, her eyes on fire, suddenly re-energized. Seeing her respond with such obvious pleasure, something inside me *unlocked.*

I'd always played sadism as service—giving masochists what they wanted. But this was different. This was me taking. Me claiming. Not because she asked. Because I wanted it. This was the edge.

And the wildest part? She wanted that too. She'd offered it to me before, but I had been too afraid of myself.

"10…"

I let the *beast* inside me step forward without shame—

"9…"

Tapped into something beyond myself—

"8…"

Let the fire in me guide my hand—

"7…"

Opened to my animal—

"6…"

I was not a monster.

"5…"

I was a god.

That was the night I let my own Dark Masculine lead—the part of me that didn't back down from intensity, the one that said: I can take you further, and you'll come out stronger. And Casey met me in her Dark Feminine—wanting more, pushing back, but also choosing to open.

Her surrender was her power.

THE CONSENT NO ONE TALKS ABOUT

Did I hesitate at that moment? No. Should I have? I knew her well enough. We'd played many times before. We were skilled at coming back into attunement with each other, never blaming each other when a line got blurry, always assuming the best of intentions because we always *had* the best of intentions.

SIDEBAR: The Self-check of the Sadist

Before stepping into a sadistic scene, ask: Is my desire rooted in presence or in power over another? Am I leading, or am I taking without care?

The Dark Masculine's strength is not in the intensity itself, but in the ability to wield intensity with precision and care, to strike deep without losing attunement.

But intensity without that kind of self-check is dangerous.

I knew a sadistic Domme who didn't check in with Herself before a scene. She was carrying heavy life stress but convinced herself She could still hold the scene with integrity. Her submissive—a man She'd played with for over a year—offered himself to Her, trusting their rhythm and their rapport. But that night, Her sadism wasn't clean, or sacred. It was distorted, resentment-driven.

He felt the undercurrent of that distortion immediately through Her whip—the displaced emotion, the edge that wasn't just sadistic but punishing. One should not underestimate the power of authentic presence…

And though he said nothing at that moment, after the scene ended, he never offered himself to Her again.

Consent is more than negotiation, more than "Yes, I want this." Consent is also self-awareness. I've spent years playing at the edges of power and surrender, giving people the experiences they craved from both the bottom and the top. But in that moment—when I took that countdown with Casey *for myself*—I felt something move: the thrill of not knowing where my own edge actually was.

HURT VERSUS HARM—THE SHADOW LINE

Every self-aware sadist asks the same question: *How do I know I won't take it too far?*

The answer is in the line between *hurt and harm.*

Hurt is intentional. *Chosen.*

Harm is *reckless.* Unconscious.

For the sadist and masochist, hurt is a sensation given in trust. Harm is power wielded without care.

Sadism in coherence is the Dark Masculine wielding intensity with precision, guiding someone to their edge and catching them there. Masochism in coherence is the Dark Feminine opening wide, demanding: *Take me further. Show me what I can hold.*

The danger isn't the desire. It's the unconsciousness.

PRACTICES OF THE SHADOW—WHERE THE BEAST SPEAKS

Different kinks give us different ways to play at this threshold. Each one is a language of sensation that teaches us where hurt ends and harm begins.

- Electroplay—Lightning on the skin, the crackle of sound as arousing as the jolt itself. Anticipation becomes the real mindfuck.
- Chastity & Orgasm Denial—The hunger stretched thin, where surrender is built from the ache of what's withheld. Desire as discipline.
- Cock & Ball Torture (CBT)—Agony and ecstasy riding the same line. Extreme trust. Extreme altered states.

Each practice is a mirror. Each one forces us to see what power really does in our bodies.

EMOTIONAL SADISM

Sadism isn't always physical. Sometimes it's emotional. Just like the body can transmute pain into pleasure, the psyche can do the same with shame, embarrassment, and degradation—if the scene is crafted with care.

Emotional sadism is a delicate art. And within it, there's a critical distinction between humiliation and degradation that many people overlook. Generally, humiliation targets an action or a response—*"What you're doing is bad,"* or *"You shouldn't be reacting like that."* It evokes embarrassment, which some of us find erotic. Humiliation as a kink is relatively common. I get turned on when someone calls out my arousal—the way my nipples betray me or my pussy swells visibly. That slight flush of shame in response to something edgy that I consider erotic? That's a sweet spot for me and my embarrassment kink.

Degradation, on the other hand, goes deeper, and is far less common. Instead of targeting the action, it targets the self: "You *are bad.* You *are less than.* You *are nothing."* It's not just emotionally risky—it's soul-level edge play. For those who crave it, it can be profoundly satisfying. But the line between hurt and harm here is razor-thin.

And even these definitions aren't absolute. The real distinction isn't written in stone—it's written in the psyche of the person receiving it. What feels like degradation to one may land as humiliation—or as pure turn-on—for another.

I know of a scene that took place in an expertly-held container at a kinky camping event—negotiated with care, held with support, and designed for deep *degradation*. The bottom knew herself and her desires intimately. She was buried up to her neck, urinated on, and verbally degraded. And she thrived in it.

Until someone smeared her makeup while she was still buried.

That single act crossed a line. Not because it was more extreme—but because, *for her*, it shifted the energy from degradation to *humiliation*. She safe-worded immediately. The scene stopped. She was held, tended to, and brought back to center gently. And while the line had been hit, what followed was a long interaction of beautiful repair that they all grew from. That's the kind of intimacy this work can generate—if all parties are prepared to meet the edge with care and deep presence.

Emotional sadism, when wielded with integrity, is just as potent as physical play. But it demands a depth of self-knowledge and trust that few people are willing to cultivate. And for some, it's the deepest form of release there is.

RECLAIMING THE BEAST

We all have a sadist inside us. Even those who swear they don't. It shows up in ways most people never recognize as sadism. The way someone relishes a sharp comment that lands just right. The way a lover teases and denies, pushing their partner to the edge of desperation. The way someone enjoys watching another squirm as a way to feel in *control.*

Sadism isn't always about pain. It's about power, and whether we admit it or not, power lives inside us all.

The work isn't in taming the beast. It's in making the beast sacred.

Sadists are threshold-keepers, inviting descent. Masochists are the sacred gates, opening the body wide. The Dark Masculine holds the strike. The Dark Feminine devours it whole.

This is erotic alchemy. The body speaks what the mind cannot name.

CLOSING THE SCENE: THE SACRED EXCHANGE

The beast is not your enemy. The lamb is not your weakness.

Sadism and masochism are sacred languages—of sensation, of longing, and of trust. The conscious sadist doesn't only take. They wield intensity with reverence. The conscious masochist doesn't only suffer. They alchemize pain into power.

This isn't pain just to hurt. It's the place where the Dark Feminine and Dark Masculine collide. And when they do, instead of destroying you, the impact changes you.

EROTIC ALCHEMY IN PRACTICE: DANCING WITH THE BEAST

Embodiment

Take two to three minutes. Let your body replay a moment you recently felt anger, frustration, or the urge to lash out. Curl your fists, grit your teeth, stomp, growl, or let a sound escape from you.

Stay with it for just a few breaths. Then pause—notice how your body feels when the energy is expressed instead of being stuffed down.

> **Spicy Add-On:** Add self-pleasure after the growl. Touch yourself while staying connected to that beast energy. Notice how the sounds or the rawness change the texture of your arousal and your pleasure.

Expression

Journal a dialogue with your inner beast. Let it speak freely: What does it want, what does it crave, what does it hate holding back? Then write as the part of you that can hold this beast responsibly. How could that same energy be channeled in ways that feel alive rather than destructive?

> **Spicy Add-On:** Write it as a fantasy scene. Let your beast describe what it would do if it could act without consequence—snarling, pinning, clawing, taking. Then, if it feels safe, read it aloud to yourself or whisper it into a recorder so you can hear your own hunger voiced.

Integration—Partnered

With a trusted person, co-create a short, negotiated scene. One of you takes the role of sadist for just a few minutes—through spanking, hair pulling, tickling, or rough grabs. The other plays masochist, leaning into the sensation without needing to pretend it's easy. Use clear start/stop words.

Take time after to debrief: What surprised you, what turned you on, what felt cathartic?

Then switch.

> **Spicy Add-On:** Let the "beast" role escalate into pursuit—one chases, pins, or snarls while the other resists before surrendering. Keep it controlled but allow it to feel primal and hot.

Integration (24-Hour Challenge)

For one day, watch when the "beast" shows up—in sarcasm, impatience, or the urge to push back. Instead of shaming it, ask: What's the coherent version of this urge? If you want to roar, coherence might look like speaking firmly without cruelty. If you want to shove, coherence might be putting that same force into movement, sport, or sex. Practice acting from this contained awareness in real time.

> **Spicy Add-On:** When you feel the beast surface in everyday life, eroticize it later in private. Replay the moment in your body—growl, snap, or reenact the stance—and then channel it straight into pleasure, either solo or partnered, letting that frustrated energy become arousal and release.

PART THREE: RELATING

LOVE AS AN ENERGY, NOT A CONTRACT

CHAPTER 9

SOVEREIGN LOVE

THE END OF CODEPENDENCY, THE BEGINNING OF CHOICE

No one tells you that choosing yourself might break your heart. That sometimes the bravest thing you'll ever do is say *no* to what's familiar. Not because you want to leave, but because staying would require you to abandon yourself.

THE OFFER TO SHRINK

We sat together in silence, though the air between us was thick with everything we weren't saying.

For years, Matt and I had been unraveling and reweaving our marriage, stretching it to accommodate a kind of freedom-in-relationship that most people never even whispered about. What had begun as sexy exploration—first with another couple and their boyfriend, then with our naughty couples pod, then with our kinky pack—had evolved into something neither of us could have predicted.

It was no longer just about sex or kink. No longer about the thrill of watching each other play, the high of exploration, or the erotic rush of possibility.

Polyamory was a deeper kind of intimacy. A deeper emotional connection. The possibility of love that stretched beyond our marriage.

And with all of that came fear.

I had been the one to first suggest opening our marriage. And yet I had also been the one who struggled the most along the journey—when my husband's desire for other women became real, when I had to sit in the uncomfortable truth of jealousy and envy, of insecurity, or of wondering whether I was enough.

It was an old story, one that started long before we met…

We'd processed all of these feelings with each other over the years again and again. Our longings. Fears. Visions for the future and for our family. My honest desire to be on the other side of my self-worth and abandonment issues.

At that time, there were no spaces to connect with people who were *relationshipping* the way we had been. No one to talk to or compare stories with, or to seek wisdom from.

That night, Matt was tired. Tired of hearing my fears out loud, tired of watching me wrestle with them. When he finally looked at me, his voice was quiet but steady.

"Maybe we should shut it all down."

The words hit my chest like a blunt force. My breath caught, and for a moment, the room tilted. It wasn't an ultimatum or a demand. It was a simple offering. A chance to step back from the ledge.

It would be easier. Simpler.

But the larger part of me—my body—was already screaming no. My chest constricted, my stomach dropped, and heat rose in my throat all at once.

I couldn't go back. I couldn't shrink. Not for him… not even for the version of us that once fit like a perfect puzzle.

I didn't hesitate. My voice came out more certain than I felt inside.

"I can't. I won't."

The words landed like a stone in still water. We both felt the ripple.

And that's when I saw it—the truth that neither of us had really said out loud:

He wasn't tired of polyamory. He was tired of *holding space for my emotions.*

And here's my own shadow: I had been asking him to do what I wasn't yet willing to do for myself. To regulate me. To reassure me. To carry the weight of feelings I hadn't learned to hold. My distorted Dark Feminine still longed to be rescued, even as my higher self was screaming for sovereignty. That looked like asking him to calm me instead of learning to calm myself.

WHERE WE FIRST LEARNED TO ABANDON OURSELVES

Most of us don't learn sovereign love in our families. We learn to manage others—how to make ourselves small so no one gets upset. To sense every shift in the room—and preemptively censor ourselves so no one explodes.

We learn that our feelings are dangerous. That our truth is too much. That love must be earned through control. And **we abandon ourselves to keep the peace.**

This is a survival mechanism.

Then we grow up. But no one teaches us how to mature *out* of that survival. Because most of the adults around us never did. So we enter relationships with the same template.

If I manage your emotions, maybe I'll be safe.
If I abandon myself, maybe I'll finally be loved.

That night with Matt, I saw the thread clearly. I wasn't just wrestling with polyamory—I was standing face-to-face with every childhood imprint. And for the first time, I chose not to disappear inside them.

Sovereign love doesn't ask you to disappear. It asks you to come back to yourself.

For so much of our marriage, we had leaned on each other in an unhealthy, emotionally codependent way, expecting the other to *do* something about our feelings when we had them. If one of us was drowning, the other was supposed to save them. If one of us was in pain, the other was supposed to *be the medicine*.

But that night, something inside me shifted.

I was done outsourcing my pain.

I can see how much of my Dark Feminine shadow was at play there—the part of me that would hand over my sovereignty just to be chosen, then secretly resent the very person I'd asked to hold it. That pattern burned through so much of my marriage before I could finally name it.

I wasn't just deciding relationships that night. I was making a decision about *who I was becoming.*

Like Persephone, I had swallowed the seeds. And I would never fully belong to the surface world again.

ALTERNATIVE STRUCTURES, DEEPER SHADOWS

So many people think polyamory will solve their boredom. That open relationships will fix their unmet desires. That kink will save their dying sex lives.

But new structures don't dissolve old wounds. They just *expose* them faster.

You can't bypass your abandonment wound by dating multiple people. You can't fix your lack of safety by calling it freedom. **You can't reach enlightenment through sex if you're using sex to escape yourself.**

In fact, all of these wounds and unresolved echoes are amplified.

Alternative relationship styles are powerful and deeply transformative—but not because they're easier. In fact, they're more complex. To be transformed, they require expanded levels of emotional honesty, a deeper capacity for self-regulation, and a willingness to sit inside the fire of your own fear without projecting it onto others.

Polyamory—or as I call it, *sovereign relating*—didn't break me, and it could have. Instead, it revealed me to myself.

Alternative relationships are a *mirror* reflecting everything you haven't yet made peace with.

Love built on sovereignty does not collapse. It does not demand. It does not manipulate.

It's not: If you loved me, you would…

It's: I love you, and I love me. Both get to exist here.

This is emotional adulthood. This is erotic maturity.

SIDEBAR: How to Spot Distortion Versus Coherence in Real Time

The Dark Feminine in distortion hints, tests, inflates or escalates urgency to be chosen.

The Dark Masculine in distortion lectures, problem-solves feelings away, or withdraws to avoid discomfort.

The Dark Feminine in coherence names the truth plainly—"I'm jealous and scared; I'm still a yes to this path."

The Dark Masculine in coherence stays present and specific—"I hear you. Here's what I can offer today; here's what I can't..."

A Simple Script:

Dark Feminine: "Here's what's true for me. Here's what I need. I can hold myself; I'm not asking you to fix it."

Dark Masculine: "I'm here. I'm not going to argue with your feelings. I can do X; I can't do Y. Does that help?"

When we stop outsourcing our emotional weather to others, we stop trying to control their choices so we feel safe. We grieve when they can't meet us, yes—but we don't abandon ourselves—or blame them—in the process. We hold our center.

This is the alchemy of sovereign love.

THE GIFT OF NOT BEING MET—BUT STILL BEING HELD

It was years later. I was still married, but my husband and I were living in different cities—he with a partner, and me on my own.

I'd been dating Justin for a year and a half when I realized something had shifted. My feelings had tipped—not just "I care about you" love, but that melt-into-someone's-ribcage kind of ache of being *in love*. And I needed to say it. To stop hiding the truth of where I was. But we hadn't used those words between us yet, so I didn't know how they would land.

One night, heart pounding, I told him. I let the words fall, unclothed: "I love you."

He breathed, and I could feel him steady himself. His eyes softened. His voice was careful, honest.

"Thank you." He paused for a moment. "I don't feel the same. I can't say it back."

Heat rushed up my neck. My chest squeezed. And still—I was calm. Because I hadn't said it to get something back. I said it because hiding it had started to feel like abandonment of myself.

I told him I wasn't asking for more time, more commitment, or anything different. I just wanted the freedom to be in my truth. He nodded. Received it. And from that moment on, I said *I love you* when I felt it, especially when we parted.

That, too, was sovereignty.

Not long after, he initiated a follow-up conversation. He was curious why it felt so difficult for him to "go there" emotionally, not just with me, but with another partner who also had deep feelings for him.

I held space for him. Reminded him I didn't need anything from him. I wondered aloud whether he was saving that part of himself for the woman he hoped to build a family with. We both knew he wanted that. He was more than a decade younger than me, and I wasn't looking to "start that clock over again" myself. It made sense that he was saving parts of himself for that.

Months later, after another date night of laughter and touch and closeness, he went to leave the next morning. But at the door, he paused. He turned back, placed his hands deliberately on my arms, and looked directly into me.

"Hey. I love you."

My heart bloomed. I beamed and said it back. Not with more weight than before, not with less—it was just as true as it had always been. I hadn't needed the words. But to be met in them? To be received without demand? It was a gift.

And I believe—maybe—he was able to share it because I'd never required it. Because I'd never needed him to be anywhere other than exactly where he was.

In that moment, he held steady—clear, present. I told the truth without apologizing for it and didn't fold when it wasn't mirrored back. Together, that polarity made the love feel free instead of forced.

CLOSING THE SCENE: THE LOVE YOU WERE MEANT FOR

Sovereign love doesn't ask you to disappear. It doesn't punish you for feeling. It doesn't require you to earn your place. It meets you where you are—because you already know how to meet yourself.

It's the quiet revolution of not needing someone else to be different for you to feel whole. It's unlearning the idea that your partner is responsible for fixing your pain.

And if someone can't meet you there, you don't chase or punish; you grieve, you breathe, and you come back to center. That's sovereign love.

EROTIC ALCHEMY IN PRACTICE: CHOOSING YOURSELF FIRST

Integration—Solo

Notice when you want reassurance or validation from someone else—a partner, a friend, a lover. Let yourself feel the sensations of that longing in your body: maybe a tightness in your chest, a pull in your stomach, or the ache of wanting to be chosen. Place one hand on your heart, one on your belly, and say aloud: *I see you. I hear you. I've got you.*

Breathe until you feel your body soften, or the sensations shift. Let the acknowledgement land in your body.

> **Spicy Add-On:** After you ground yourself, turn that longing into touch. Self-pleasure slowly while repeating the words: *I choose you. I choose me.* Let your body feel what it's like to soothe the ache with your own hands and arousal, not by reaching outward.

Integration—Partnered

Invite someone into a mirroring exercise. Stand or sit facing each other. Each of you names aloud one desire you've held back—big or small. The other responds with acknowledgment, not solutions: *I hear you. Thank you for trusting me with that.*

Switch roles. Notice how being witnessed without fixing changes the way the longing feels.

> **Spicy Add-On:** Make it erotic. Each of you shares a hidden erotic desire—what you fantasize about, what you

crave, what you've been too shy to name. The partner listens without judgment, maybe even with a hand on your body for grounding. Let the arousal build in the tension of being seen without the immediate fulfillment.

Integration (24-Hour Challenge)

For the next day, notice when envy or comparison arises—maybe a friend is praised instead of you, your partner desires someone else, or you see someone radiate a quality you long for. Instead of thinking, *They have it and I don't,* pause.

Write or whisper: *That quality lives in me too.* If you see their confidence, claim your own. If you see their freedom, name the ways yours already exists. Treat it not as a lack but as a mirror calling something forward in you.

Spicy Add-On: At the end of the day, take one of those qualities you noticed in someone else—confidence, sensuality, freedom—and embody it in erotic play. Dress, move, or touch yourself as if you *are* that quality. If with a lover, act it out for them: Let them see the version of you that already owns it.

CHAPTER 10

WHEN FANTASY MEETS TABOO

OWNING THE STORIES THAT TURN YOU ON

Kinks and fetishes don't emerge from nowhere. They're not random, broken, or perverse. They're stories etched into our cells. Some were written before we had language. Some are passed down through ancestry. Some are carved into us by trauma, while others arrive like whispers from other lifetimes.

Sometimes, we never find out their root—and that's okay. I used to think I had to trace every kink back to its origin, but over time I realized **the mystery itself is part of the medicine.** The task isn't always to explain, but to meet what's emerging with reverence instead of judgment.

Every urge holds power, whether or not we can trace its history. The invitation is to stop judging the shape of desire and start listening to what it's pointing us toward.

THE MAN WHO FOUND POWER IN PAIN

Early in my kink journey, a professional Domme shared a story about a client whose request startled even Her. She had a client who, in every session, asked Her to stand across the room in high heels, charge at him with full force, and kick him in the balls.

I remember saying: *Help me understand.*

Years before, the man had been mugged in an alley by two men and a woman. The men pinned his arms while the woman was ordered to kick him in the balls, before they robbed him. But when the kick landed, instead of collapsing in pain, his body surged with raw power. Energy shot up his spine, his arms broke free, and it awakened something primal in him. He fought off his attackers, then turned to the woman who had kicked him and growled, "You'd better run."

And she did.

This moment was imprinted on him not as trauma, but as *power*. His body coded it as strength. Pain had been the ignition switch for his power. His survival. His victory.

Later, he tried a myriad of ways to recreate that experience on his own but couldn't make it work. So he turned to a professional and, in a controlled, consensual way, turned a moment of forced helplessness into chosen surrender. Every kick was a ritual that reconnected him to his Dark Masculine—his resilience, his fight, his breakthrough.

That is the shadow's secret: Sometimes what looks like perversion is really power, remembered.

REWIRING MY ORGASM

For most of my life, I couldn't reach orgasm without fantasy. I needed elaborate, often taboo scenarios in my head—restraint, forced pleasure, power imbalance. No matter what was happening in reality, my climax lived in an imagined *elsewhere*.

I didn't question it for decades. In fact, I carried a lot of shame around it. I thought it was just how my body worked. But as I deepened into my erotic sovereignty, I realized something:

My orgasms had been programmed.

As age five, I had experienced regular sexual abuse at a babysitter's home, and then at age six, incest at home. I learned to disassociate from my body, escaping into imagination while my body endured what it had no language for. Fantasy became *survival*. It bridged sensation and safety. And even decades later, that bridge was still the only way my body trusted pleasure.

But sovereignty meant something else. It meant choosing arousal from presence rather than from escape. I write about this in more detail in *Flesh & Flame: Pleasure as the Portal to Divine Mastery,* but the roots of my fantasy dependency weren't random.

That's why reclaiming it mattered so deeply. I wasn't just rewiring my orgasm—I was rewriting what it meant to be safe in my body.

I used physical and mental practices to disconnect my orgasm from fantasy. As I self-pleasured, I started ceasing the fantasy just before climax, gradually lengthening the time I cut it off—until one day, I didn't need fantasy at all. My body was re-attuned to itself. My physical pleasure was *mine* again.

But I need to be honest—I didn't always succeed. Sometimes I fell back into fantasy because it felt easier than facing my own body. My distorted Dark Masculine wanted control because it was safer to stay in my head than risk the raw, unpredictable truth of my body.

That's the work of the Dark Feminine and Dark Masculine together: She insists the shame and secrecy be faced. He holds steady so the body can relearn what safety feels like.

Together, they rewire what once felt broken into a new coherence.

Rewiring my orgasm for presence instead of escape was one of the most powerful reclamations I've ever made. And it showed me something most people never talk about:

Fetishes can shift.

Erotic imprinting is not fixed.

Trauma evolves when we meet it with conscious, loving awareness.

This didn't mean I no longer enjoyed fantasizing or restraints or forced orgasm. It meant those **desires became choices rather than needs** because I had finally transcended the original entanglement.

These are the doorways of the Dark Feminine and the Dark Masculine. Kinks and fetishes aren't simple indulgences—they're often a part of you that was exiled.

MY KINKS: THE THEME OF DESIRE

While the need dissolved, the kinks remained. This isn't a full list of my kinks by any means, but what I've noticed is a theme: Desire itself turns me on.

- *Bulge/Nipple kink*—The outline of desire itself, visible and undeniable.
- *Voyeurism*—Watching people bask in their pleasure, which gives me permission to lean into mine.
- *Bondage*—Probably my favorite. This can be physical restraints like cuffs, being held down, or bound with rope, or it can be mental restraints like predicament play, edging, or orgasm denial.
- *Worship*—The devotion kink. Being adored, exalted, or placed on a pedestal—for simply *being*. Someone acknowledging the reverence of my body, my energy, and my presence as holy. And yes, offering that reverence to another in return, when there is true attunement. Worship is not about status. It's about a deep, energetic presence and the amplification of awe.
- *Power imbalance*—Programming from childhood, reshaped and reclaimed in my adulthood to include other imbalanced power hierarchies.

What once felt like shame had become a map. My body was never trying to punish me with these desires. It was *trying to help me reclaim them*.

My desires, once untouchable without shame or pain, became the very things I sought. And **this is where we separate programming from self-mastery.**

From fear, need, and shame… to desire, choice, and sovereignty.

PROGRAMMING VS. SELF-MASTERY—UNDERSTANDING THE SOURCE OF DESIRE

Not every kink is trauma. Not every fantasy needs decoding. But erotic sovereignty means asking:

- Is this desire mine, or was it conditioned into me?
- Does it expand me, or keep me locked in repetition?
- If I had the power to rewrite my erotic blueprint, would I choose it again?

These are the questions that bring power to our pleasure. Because pleasure is not just about chasing sensation. It's about choosing how we engage with it.

When the Dark Feminine rises, she says: *Feed me. Stop starving this hunger.* When the Dark Masculine stands beside her, he says: *I can hold it. Bring it all.*

Together, they turn what once felt taboo into a doorway.

THE SCIENCE OF EROTIC IMPRINTING

Science calls it imprinting. Pleasure paired with a trigger creates a pattern:

Pleasure + Sensory Trigger = Desire

Fear + Sensory Trigger = Kink

Power + Sensory Trigger = Fetish

Sometimes the pattern is clear. Sometimes it makes no sense. That's because some desires aren't born of this life. They are soul-level. They arrive without explanation, only resonance. The first time I felt worship as arousing, it didn't come from trauma. It came like a memory. Something ancient in me remembered being honored as divine. That wasn't pathology. That was truth resurfacing.

Not every shadow is brokenness.

And when you begin using your taboos as erotic medicine, the line between pleasure, fear, and power blur...

CLOSING THE SCENE: YOUR DESIRES ARE SACRED

Your desires are not random. They are maps. Some were written by wounds. Some were inherited from bloodlines. Some are echoes of lifetimes you don't consciously recall.

But every one of them points toward your power.

The work is not to fix them. The work is to honor them. To listen. To choose. Because when you stop fearing your erotic shadows—and start honoring them—you begin the work of becoming whole.

EROTIC ALCHEMY IN PRACTICE: OWNING THE STORIES THAT TURN YOU ON

Embodiment

Bring to mind a fantasy you return to often. Play it out in your imagination just far enough to feel your body respond—heat, pulse, breath. Then pause. Ask yourself: *Do I actually want to live this in real life, or do I want it to stay fantasy fuel?*

Notice the difference.

> **Spicy Add-On:** Touch yourself while you imagine a well-remembered fantasy. Let your arousal rise with the fantasy. Sit in the heat of wanting without rushing to release, just to see what it feels like to hold the charge.

Expression

Write the fantasy down. Then add: *If I could choose this freely, without shame or story, how would I want to embody it now?* Maybe you keep the fantasy only on paper. Maybe you act out a piece of it alone. Maybe you recognize it's not something you want to do but love to dream about. All are valid.

> **Spicy Add-On:** Read your fantasy out loud—to yourself in the mirror, recorded on your phone, or to a trusted partner. Notice how your body reacts to hearing it spoken instead of written.

Integration (24-Hour Challenge)

For one day, track when a fantasy or craving pops into your mind. Instead of pushing it away, pause and name it. Ask:

Is this desire mine today, or is it old programming? Do I want to keep this one alive or let it dissolve?

> **Spicy Add-On:** At the end of the day, pick one fantasy that showed up and give it a small, embodied nod: Dress in a way that matches its energy, strike a pose, or self-pleasure with that image in mind. Not the whole fantasy—just a taste.

Integration—Partnered

Share one piece of a fantasy with someone you trust. Don't jump into acting it out yet—just speak it out loud. Let your Dark Feminine voice name the hunger without apology. Let the Dark Masculine voice stay grounded, present, and non-reactive as it's received. Notice how simply speaking desire shifts the charge.

> **Spicy Add-On:** With clear negotiation, act out a piece of a fantasy together. Keep it short and deliberate—five minutes of roleplay, a single scene, one detail.
>
> Then debrief together: What turned you on, what felt flat, what surprised you? This isn't about performance; it's about letting the body taste what the mind has been holding.

CHAPTER 11

CONSENSUAL NON-CONSENT

THE MOST DANGEROUS TRUST

There is a moment in certain kinds of play—a flash of tension or struggle—where the lines between resistance and surrender blur. Where the body betrays the mind. Where words say *no* while breath and pulse whisper *more.*

This is the heart of Consensual Non-Consent (CNC): the illusion of force. The edge where power and trust meet so fiercely that they dissolve into one another.

At its best, CNC isn't about force at all. It's about the Dark Masculine holding such an unwavering presence that the one surrendering can finally stop bracing. It's about the Dark Feminine roaring through the body, demanding to be claimed, devoured, overwhelmed. And it's about both partners consenting to the illusion of chaos, knowing the container underneath is rock solid. CNC is energy exchange at its most primal—where one partner "loses control" in their hunger, and the other is taken, ravished, or claimed in a way that feels unfiltered and electrifying.

But CNC is also one of the most misunderstood, misused, and *dangerous* edges in kink. When wielded without care, it's not play—it's harm. Which is why this particular doorway requires more responsibilities, more self-awareness, and more communication than almost any other.

THE THRILL OF BEING TAKEN

CNC carries a charge unlike anything else.

Like primal play, it often builds in a crescendo: the teasing, the chase, the inevitability of capture. What ignites me most in these scenes is not simply being "taken," but feeling like my desire has awakened something so feral in my partner that they *can't* hold back. That their hunger consumes them.

To be wanted that deeply is intoxicating.

But here is the paradox: I chose it. I invited the scene. I gave my consent to lose my consent. And in that, CNC becomes an act of devotion.

CNC is not about force—it is about trust so deep that the illusion of force becomes safe.

When done well, I don't just surrender to my partner's desire—they surrender to it, too. They stop performing control and let themselves be undone by their own hunger. That's the paradox most people miss: CNC isn't about losing power. It's about wielding power so exquisitely that both partners can dissolve into it.

WHEN FANTASY BECOMES DANGER

I once was in a dynamic with a Dominant, Troy, who understood my love of power imbalance. He could push my buttons with a whisper, arouse me into submission with the smallest gesture. One day, He suggested staging a CNC scene where He would break into my house and "take me."

Part of me was aroused. And part of me froze. Because this wasn't just roleplay. It brushed too close to the truth of my childhood trauma—abuse and violation I had no choice in. To recreate it physically would not have been arousing; it would have been retraumatizing.

That distinction—between fantasy and reality—is everything. Some desires are meant to stay in the erotic imagination, where they are hot, thrilling, and safe. Others can be safely embodied. The wisdom is in knowing the difference.

And it wasn't just about me or my past. He was *too* sadistic for me to consent to this. I would later come to learn just how important that decision was. Because while Troy never forced me into anything, there was a moment where He chose to treat my body's response as a yes, even though my words and energy were loudly saying no. That wasn't a "miscommunication." It was a failure of attunement.

And it's not just about words. At that time, when I was in a submissive state, I was in a vulnerable, childlike mental space, which made sense considering the context of our form of play. But when I was in that state, I didn't have the same confidence, the same courage, or the same clarity as my bold, everyday self because *she*—the younger self who had been sexually abused—was the one who was surfacing. Not the adult, integrated me.

Which meant I wasn't fully in control of my own headspace.

This was my own distortion showing. I told myself I was sovereign, but the truth was, part of me wanted to hand over responsibility so I wouldn't have to face my own yes or no. That was my Dark Feminine in collapse—giving up from fear rather than opening from desire.

I had let *her* give too much of *my* power away.

This set me up for harm. This was a crucial lesson for me in understanding the psychological states that can emerge in BDSM play.

I knew a woman, a rope bottom, who went nonverbal in subspace when she was tied, but who refused to tell her rope Tops about this because she was afraid They would refuse to tie her. What's worse: She was severely hard of hearing and sometimes removed her hearing aids altogether for a scene, making the danger for everyone involved more acute.

This wasn't just risky. It was manipulative.

She was consciously abdicating responsibility for her physical, emotional, and mental safety onto Someone Else without getting their explicit consent first.

A person who does this is a danger to play with.

LEARNING FROM EDGES

Sometimes, we don't know our edges until we cross them. That's part of the work.

I've had scenes where the aftercare was messy because something hit a nerve I hadn't anticipated. That doesn't always mean someone did something wrong. But it does mean something important was revealed.

The mark of a safe partner is not perfection. It's responsiveness. It's the Top who pauses even when you say you're "fine." It's the bottom who admits, *I crossed my own line, and I need help integrating.*

Edges are inevitable. What matters is whether we meet them with awareness—or with denial.

WHEN SAFE WORDS ARE WAIVED

There are those who play even deeper: "no safe word" scenes, sometimes called Total Power Exchange (TPE).

People waive their safe word for many reasons. Sometimes it's because the trust is so deep that words aren't needed. Sometimes it's because they want to be pushed past their own limits, or because full surrender itself feels devotional.

But it's also dangerous. Some do it to prove themselves, to impress a Dom, or because they don't feel worthy of boundaries. That's when it's reckless.

What Makes It Safe?

- Only engaging in TPE with Someone who has earned that level of trust.
- Establishing nonverbal signals that still express an edge (a double tap, dropping a small object, etc.).
- Making it reversible—even in a full surrender scene, there must be a way to re-negotiate later.

It's one of the riskiest agreements possible. Waiving a safe word without deep trust and calibration is reckless.

Done in coherence, TPE can be transcendent. Done in distortion, it can destroy trust permanently.

The deeper the surrender, the deeper the *mutual responsibility.*

SIDEBAR: Dark Feminine & Dark Masculine in CNC—Distortion vs. Coherence

Dark Feminine in Distortion

- *Collapses into fear and calls it surrender.*
- *Hands away responsibility, hoping to be rescued.*
- *Says "yes" when her body or heart means "no."*

Dark Feminine in Coherence

- *Chooses surrender as an act of devotion.*
- *Names her limits honestly, then offers herself fully.*
- *Lets her hunger roar, trusting it will be met with steadiness.*

Dark Masculine in Distortion

- *Mistakes the body's reaction for consent.*
- *Plays out their own shadow or stress through "intensity."*
- *Ignores signals in order to stay in control.*

Dark Masculine in Coherence

- *Holds presence so steady the Feminine can stop bracing.*
- *Listens for the truth beneath the words and the body.*
- *Wields power with precision, never recklessness.*

CLOSING THE SCENE—CNC AS THE ULTIMATE EDGE OF TRUST

CNC is not about violence or humiliation or about being broken down. It is about the mastery of power and surrender.

It's about building a container so strong that the illusion of danger becomes safe enough to step into.

It's about power wielded with such clarity that fear alchemizes into ecstasy. About surrender so deep that both partners are consumed by deep trust.

CNC is the razor's edge of erotic alchemy. It demands responsibility, honesty, and mastery. But when it is met with that level of consciousness, it becomes more than kink. It becomes a doorway into the Mystery itself—where fear, hunger, and devotion collide, and both partners come out changed.

EROTIC ALCHEMY IN PRACTICE: PLAYING WITH POWER AND PERMISSION

Embodiment

Close your eyes and recall a time you felt a mix of fear and desire—your pulse quickened, your breath caught, and yet part of you leaned toward it. Let yourself sit with that tension. Notice how your body holds both signals at once.

> **Spicy Add-On**: While holding that memory, press your own wrists gently against a wall, bed, or chair—as if restrained. Or imagine doing that to someone else. Breathe into the mix of fear and heat that rises.

Integration—Solo

Write down a fantasy that edges into CNC territory. Circle the parts that feel hot. Underline the parts that feel unsafe or tied to old wounds. This helps you separate the fuel from the danger—what belongs in fantasy, and what could be safe in play.

> **Spicy Add-On:** Read your fantasy aloud in a whisper—into a mirror, or even just under your breath. Let your body feel what happens when the words leave your head and enter the room.

Integration—Partnered

With someone you trust, set up a *short* roleplay. One plays the pursuer, the other the pursued. Use voice, presence, and light touch—but keep the frame clear: This is play, and either of you can stop it anytime.

Switch roles if you like.

Spicy Add-On: Add one layer—gentle pinning of wrists, a hand over the mouth with clear signals, or the sound of a door closing behind you. Keep it short and deliberate. The heat is in the illusion, not escalation.

SIDEBAR: Safety Standards for CNC

- *Use a safe word (or clear nonverbal signal if you might go nonverbal).*
- *Negotiate what is on the table and what is absolutely not.*
- *Agree on how to pause the scene if it feels off.*
- *Build slowly. Start light. Debrief after.*

Integration (24-Hour Challenge)

For the next day, notice where you surrender your "no" in everyday life—agreeing to something you don't want, staying quiet when you'd rather speak. In those moments, practice saying a simple, clear no out loud. It could be "No thanks, I'm not available," "I'd rather not," or even just "No." The point isn't the size of the situation—it's teaching your body and voice that your no is safe, valid, and allowed. Strengthening this muscle outside of play makes CNC safer inside of it.

Spicy Add-On: If you're ready for more, negotiate a CNC scene with your partner that includes specific limits and signals. Examples: a pursuer who pins you against a wall while you resist, or being held down with playful force. Agree on aftercare before you begin. The point is not to erase your no, but to create a container so strong that you can choose to let go inside it.

CHAPTER 12

THE TWIN FLAME ILLUSION

CHOOSING POWER OVER DESTINY

We are fed a lie from the moment we enter this world. Nearly every fairy tale, film, book, song, and dating sim tells us that it is our life's purpose to find *The One*. Our missing piece. Our perfect match. The soul mate. The twin flame.

The mythology has been rebranded with spiritual language and dressed up as destiny. But at its core, it's still the same trap: the belief that you are incomplete without being coupled.

You are not here to find The One. You are here to *become* The One.

And when you do, you unlock the highest level of connection because you remember that you are already whole within yourself. When you realize that *separation is an illusion*, everything shifts. The love you were looking for has always been you.

INITIATION BY TWIN FLAME

When I met him, it was like being struck by lightning underwater.

Everything in me surged awake—my pussy, my heart, my voice, my knowing… It wasn't just an attraction. This was *recognition*. Soul-deep, dimension-spanning recognition. Like my entire body remembered him before my mind could catch up.

Even before his knock landed on the door, I could feel him. I didn't know what to make of the blur of sensations—this was early in my awakening journey, before I understood how to track and master my field. I was still a beginner, unpracticed in holding my own power.

We both felt it. The thunderclap. The destiny of it.

Within weeks, we were flooded with visions—past lives, battles fought side by side as winged beings of light, parallel timelines collapsing into this one. It was mythic—like something I would've written into my comic books, except this time, it wasn't fiction. I'd remembered past lives with others around me before. But this? This was something else altogether.

And the synchronicities were undeniable. He and his spouse were kinky and practiced non-monogamy. That alone felt like divine orchestration. We were both seekers, both devoted to magic and expansion. Finally—*finally*—I had met someone who could match me in vibration, magic, and intensity. A true peer.

We activated each other's gifts, triggered spontaneous downloads, and cracked open dormant codes. He was the first healer I'd met since my awakening who could actually meet me without collapsing under the weight of the spiritual lineages I carry. We even set aside romance to prioritize our energetic expansion. That's how powerful it was. That's how sure we were that something big was unfolding.

People hate hearing this, but the twin flame journey isn't about romance. It's about purification. And the stronger the pull, the sharper the fire. Because this kind of connection burns everything that isn't truth.

He brought all my core wounds to the surface. Rejection. Abandonment. Unworthiness. I alchemized them, again and again. Because I knew that was *the mirror's* purpose.

But still, I lost myself. I began to believe the story. That he was the destiny instead of the *initiation*. This was my Dark Feminine in shadow—I lost myself in the intensity, letting the hunger swallow me whole.

And then one day it abruptly ended. He messaged me to say he felt addicted to me, terrified that he was abandoning his family. And then—he disappeared. No ritual. No repair.

The fallout hit me hard. I shut down completely. I stopped meditating. Stopped creating Goddess Nights for myself. Stopped pampering myself in ritual. It was all I could do to lick my wounds and rebuild from the inside out.

The hardest part wasn't losing him. I realized how much of myself I had set aside trying to make room for a relationship that could never hold me.

And here's my accountability: I abandoned myself first.

My Dark Feminine shadow gave up her center just to be seen. My Dark Masculine drifted into fantasy instead of offering structure.

His leaving hurt, but what hurt more was seeing my own reflection in that collapse.

THE MEDICINE OF THE MIRROR

I don't blame him. He chose fear over fire. Safety over growth. I had chosen that myself, repeatedly, throughout my life.

The gift was seeing the truth: Sovereign love does not demand sacrifice. True alignment does not require a war. Sacred union doesn't starve you.

The coherent Dark Feminine rose in me then—not as the desperate girl begging to be chosen, but as the force who remembers *I am the choice.*

What he gave me was the exact medicine I needed: abandonment as the ignition point for sovereignty. He wasn't the destination. He was the fire that cracked me open.

I called my power back. I turned back to myself. Became my own sanctuary, my own Divine Counterpart.

I now know what coherent Dark Masculine would look like. Distorted, he called me an addiction—as if my presence, my fire, or our chemistry was the problem. But the truth was simpler: He couldn't hold his own intensity, so he blamed mine.

The coherent Dark Masculine doesn't vanish when the fire grows—whether it's mine, his, or the current between us. He doesn't collapse, demonize, or run. He stays. He meets heat with breath, with presence, with devotion. He holds steady, not by extinguishing the flame, but by becoming the structure strong enough for it to burn brighter.

THE PATH BACK TO SOVEREIGNTY

Twin flames aren't your perfect other half. They are *mirrors.* They show you *where you're still fragmented,* and where you still abandon yourself.

Every trigger is an invitation:

Where are you still outsourcing your worth?
Where are you waiting to be chosen instead of choosing yourself?
Where are you confusing intensity with truth?

The Dark Feminine doesn't beg to be chosen. She remembers *she is the choice.* The true Dark Masculine doesn't vanish when things get hard. He meets her depth with structure and grounded devotion.

That was the hardest mirror to face. I had already been teaching sovereignty for years, and still, I let myself forget. I abandoned my own center for a story that felt bigger than me, and the shame of that almost hurt more than losing him.

You are The One. You are the home.

CLOSING THE SCENE: TWIN FLAMES ARE PORTALS, NOT HOMES

True sacred union doesn't begin when someone else chooses you. It begins when you choose yourself—fully, fiercely, and without condition.

And from that wholeness, your Divine Counterparts arrive—not to rescue you, but to *meet* you. To *reflect your radiance.*

If it feels like a war, it's not your home.

If it asks you to shrink, it's not love.

If it blinds you to your center, it's not your destination.

Every loss is a redirection. Every rejection, a recalibration. It's a sacred whisper from the universe, saying:

Not this. Not yet. Not in this form.

The twin flame is not your ending. It's your initiation.

A portal you walk through.

And on the other side, you meet the only one who ever truly mattered: yourself.

EROTIC ALCHEMY IN PRACTICE: SOVEREIGN LOVE OVER DESTINY

Embodiment

Think of someone you've felt magnetically pulled toward—a person who lit you up but also stirred fear or insecurity. Close your eyes and feel the pull in your body. Where do you tighten? Where do you expand? Let yourself notice both the thrill and the wobble—how attraction can awaken hunger *and* destabilization at once.

> **Spicy Add-On:** Place one hand on your chest and the other between your legs. Breathe into both. Feel how attraction often sparks tenderness *and* raw desire in the same body. Let yourself rock gently or sigh, noticing how the two currents fuel one another.

Integration—Solo

Recall a time you lost your center in a relationship. Where did you hand over your worth, your truth, or your choices? Write it down honestly.

Then, write the reframe: What would staying sovereign have looked like in that moment? How would your body, words, or choices have shifted if you hadn't abandoned yourself?

> **Spicy Add-On***:* Write an alternate version as an erotic scene. Imagine yourself voicing desire without apology, holding your boundary with clarity, and letting in-

timacy or sex be hot, playful, or reverent without collapsing your sovereignty. Let your body feel the charge of that possibility as you write.

Integration—Partnered

With someone you trust, share one way a past relationship revealed a wound or shadow to you. Ask that person to reflect back the sovereignty they see in you now. Practice receiving the mirror without deflecting or downplaying.

Spicy Add-On: If you're with a lover, name one hunger that used to make you hold back or silence yourself. Then let them place a hand on your chest, kiss you, or touch you while reflecting your sovereignty. Feel the difference between being met in old wounding versus being met in your erotic power.

Integration (24-Hour Challenge)

For the next day, notice when you long to be "chosen" by someone—at work, in friendship, in intimacy. Instead of reaching outward, pause and ask yourself: How can I choose *me* here?

Take one action, however small, that affirms your own worth.

Spicy Add-On: Choose yourself *with your body.* Let yourself touch where you ache to be touched, whisper what you want to hear, or stand in front of a mirror and name your hunger aloud. Claim your own desire as valid and alive, even if no one else is there to meet it.

PART FOUR: EMBODIMENT

MASTERING PLEASURE AS A PORTAL

CHAPTER 13

BREAKING THE LAST TABOO

EROTIC ALCHEMY AS SPIRITUAL MASTERY

Pleasure is a technology. A system upgrade. A reprogramming of the deepest layers of who you are.

For centuries, society has tried to convince us that pleasure should be rationed. Hidden. Kept under control. Why? Because when someone fully owns their pleasure, something dangerous happens.

They become free.

There is nothing more threatening to systems of control than a person who cannot be shamed out of their ecstasy. Once you realize that your pleasure is not a sin, but a *source code*—a blueprint for power and self-mastery—you stop asking for permission.

You become the author of your own reality.

This is the technology they never wanted you to learn. And it's time to rewire everything you thought you knew.

PERMISSION GRANTED

Some lovers invite you to take more pleasure, to go deeper, or to open wider. But Scott, with his sweet, unapologetic hedonism, didn't just encourage me. He gave me permission.

Other lovers had wanted me to unleash sexually, to give them the full spectrum of my desire. And I believed they all meant it. But with Scott, I didn't have to *try* to open. It happened naturally *because he was already there*—so devoted to his own pleasure that mine could spill out freely, without restraint. His presence created a permission field so vast that I could bring pieces of myself I hadn't even known were missing.

He wasn't just a beautiful and generous lover. What made it different was the chemistry—raw hunger, an untamed need that had to be fed before anything else. Whenever we saw each other, skin had to find skin first—clothes pulled aside, mouths colliding, hips pressed. Only after that kind of primal claim could we even think about what came next.

And when we met in that rawness, it didn't feel like "just sex." It felt like a *return to myself.*

What made it different wasn't just heat—it was the absence of shame. He never questioned my insatiability, never flinched when my overstimulation kink took me to places other partners couldn't handle. There was no hierarchy of desires, no measure of "enough." He treated every hunger as valid, met every wave with celebration.

And so, with him, I didn't just open. I devoured. I let myself take *all* I wanted.

This, I later realized, was the Dark Feminine in her coherence—the part of me that demanded nothing yet commanded everything simply by existing without apology. And Scott's unmoving presence? That was the coherent Dark Masculine—a current that didn't try to control me but held the container steady so that I could erupt, overflow, and be fully witnessed.

THE DIVINE WITNESS: WATCHING MY INNER CHILD TAKE HER PLEASURE

The most profound moment of all came when the unhealed girl inside me—the one once taught to be ashamed of her arousal—stepped forward.

It wasn't planned. Days before, during self-pleasure, I'd had a strange thought: *What if I invited her to feel this ecstasy with me?* Not to comfort her. Or protect her. But to let her be the one taking pleasure.

It was surreal. I could feel her presence—not as a memory or a wound, but as a living pulse inside me. And my body simply knew what to do. My touch became her touch. My moans carried her voice. For the first time, she wasn't silenced. She was alive in her own desire.

And then, with Scott, it happened again.

I was on top of him, riding slowly, grinding my hips deep into his with deliberate rhythm. His size filled me perfectly, every thrust met with long waves of heat that rippled through my body. I knew he could feel my slightest response. He matched me stroke for stroke, patient and torturous, letting me build without rushing.

His hunger felt like an offering. His eyes stayed on me—fixed and reverent, almost worshipful.

And suddenly, *she* was there. Wanting to feel and be felt. Wanting to be a part of the pleasure.

I didn't push her away. I didn't override the moment with logic. I let her take.

I let her grind down harder, hips circling with hunger, voice unfiltered as moans turned guttural. My thighs trembled from the force of claiming what was once forbidden.

Scott didn't need to know the details. He didn't need to be told that he was witnessing an integration decades in the making. His only job was to stay present. To be the anchor. To feel my every contraction and surge, and not look away.

My movements deepened, my hips grinding into his even harder, owning the moment *and myself* in a way I never had before. There was nothing to hide, nothing to filter. It was both sweet and voracious.

And he was perfect for it. Because he wasn't just a lover—he was a worshiper of women's pleasure. His body was a temple of devotion, and his greatest desire when we were together was to feel me take mine.

At that moment, I felt the shift. An internal recoding. Orgasm became more than climax. It was a *carrier wave for alchemy*. **Source rewriting itself** inside me.

I felt the old programs dissolve—the ones that once whispered:

"Your arousal is dangerous."

"Your pleasure is wrong."

"You should be ashamed of how your body responds."

Gone. Burned out of my body by the flame of my climax.

And the girl—the one who had carried that shame for decades—melted into me. Not buried. Not silenced. Reclaimed.

My imprisoned power returned.

ORGASM AS THE CARRIER WAVE OF HIEROS GAMOS

Orgasmic energy is not just sensation—it is metaphysical physics. A *vibrational collapse point* where timelines shift, where the nervous system recalibrates to a new frequency, and where the ego dissolves into something vast.

This is why orgasm has been at the center of sacred rituals for millennia.

In Hieros Gamos—the sacred union of Self, Other, and All—pleasure is not reward. It is a vehicle. It is the wave that fuses chaos with order, Dark Feminine with Dark Masculine, self with Source.

In orgasm, we're not just human. We're Gods, reprogramming the universe itself. Every surge of pleasure is an activation. Every climax is an act of transmutation. And the deeper we surrender to this truth, the more we become aligned with our highest frequency of being.

WHEN THE BODY ISN'T READY

Not every orgasm has felt like power. There were times I reached edges my nervous system couldn't yet hold.

Moments when a lover fucked me through my orgasm and instead of leaning into bliss, I panicked or retreated into silence. Not because I wasn't safe—but because I still didn't feel entitled to that much aliveness.

Other times, in play party spaces, I let myself erupt fully only to collapse afterward in waves of shame. My hunger, my "too muchness," felt like a liability. Lovers recoiled, and I shrank.

These moments left residue. Whispers of my old programming: *Maybe you are too much.*

And yet, these were sacred, too. They showed me where my edges lived. Where alchemy was waiting. If I'd been brave enough to return to those moments—to hold myself at the threshold until the fear and intensity was resolved—they would've become portals.

Because erotic alchemy doesn't only happen in bliss. It happens when you stand at the edge of retreat and whisper: *I choose to stay.*

THE SACRED FORMULA OF EROTIC ALCHEMY

Erotic alchemy is the practice of transmuting raw sensation into awakening. Its formula is simple but profound:

Activation—Awakening energy through pleasure, breath, sensation, or taboo (anything that triggers an electric charge in the body).

Amplification—Holding and circulating this energy instead of dissipating it. Most people get stuck here, chasing peak pleasure without integration.

Transmutation—Directing the energy with intention, using pleasure as a vehicle for *rewiring reality*: physically, emotionally, and spiritually.

Every orgasm becomes a system upgrade. Every climax, a rewrite.

This is why pleasure has been so deeply shamed—because it is the most direct technology of liberation.

CLOSING THE SCENE: PLEASURE AS POWER

Orgasm is not just a high; it's a *system upgrade.*

Each wave of ecstasy is your body dissolving old programs and coding in new ones. Each moan, each contraction, is your power returning.

This is why they tried to control it. This is why they told you it was dirty, dangerous, or wrong.

Because when you stop apologizing for your pleasure, you stop asking permission to exist.

You don't need to consume pleasure. **You are pleasure.**

You do not chase ecstasy. You embody it.

And once you do—once you let orgasm become the fire that rewrites you—there is no going back.

This is erotic alchemy.

This is mastery.

EROTIC ALCHEMY IN PRACTICE: PLEASURE AS POWER

Embodiment

Choose a form of touch that brings you pleasure—stroking your arm, circling your hips, or running your fingers across your lips. Slow it down. Breathe with the sensation instead of rushing it. Notice how even small waves of pleasure can expand when you stay present.

> **Spicy Add-On**: Try touching yourself somewhere you normally avoid outside of sex—your inner thigh, lower back, nipples, or the hollow of your neck. Let the surprise of new territory wake your body in fresh ways.

Expression

Take a few minutes to write as if you're letting your Dark Feminine voice speak directly to you. What does she want right now—from life, from others, from you? Maybe she wants more touch, more freedom, more play, or simply to be heard without judgment.

Then, answer from your Dark Masculine voice. Instead of lofty promises, name something *tangible* he can do to steady or support that energy. It might sound like: *I'll put the phone away and run you a hot bath.* Or *I can't give you three hours tonight, but I can sit with you for twenty minutes and be fully here.*

> **Spicy Add-On:** Write this dialogue as if it's sexting with yourself. Let the Dark Feminine ask for pleasure

in explicit, turned-on language, and let the Dark Masculine respond with grounded but arousing direction.

Integration—Solo

Choose a time for self-pleasure but shift the goal from climax to pleasure exploration. Begin touching yourself in whatever way feels good until you notice your body responding—heat building in your pelvis, a pulsing in your clitoris or cock, a swelling, a wetness, a tingling under your skin. That is the energy you're working with.

When you feel that charge gathering, pause before you peak. Close your eyes. Inhale slowly through your nose and imagine that arousal moving up from your pelvis into your chest. Exhale through your mouth and let it spread—down your arms, into your legs, through your whole body.

Do this a few times. Notice how the arousal changes—sometimes it gets stronger, sometimes it softens, sometimes it spreads in waves. Place a hand over your heart or belly and whisper: *This is my power. I choose where it flows.*

If orgasm happens, notice the wave as it moves through you. If it doesn't, notice the tingling, warmth, or aliveness that lingers. Stay with it for a few minutes before moving on.

The point isn't release. It's learning that erotic energy can expand, circulate, and nourish your whole body—even without climax.

Spicy Add-On: Use a toy and lube to edge yourself several times without release. Each time you stop, breathe the arousal into another part of your body. When you finally choose to let go (if you do), let the climax feel like a full-body eruption, not just a release between your legs.

Integration—Partnered

With someone you trust, practice slowing down your pleasure together. One of you receives while the other keeps the pace deliberate, focusing on breath and presence instead of rushing. Notice how the current builds differently when you stretch it out.

Swap roles if you wish.

> **Spicy Add-On:** Agree to a "no climax" window—sixty minutes of touch, oral, or penetration without release. Let the ache build and stretch, then notice how your desire sharpens when it's not immediately satisfied.

Integration (24-Hour Challenge)

For one day, treat every burst of delight—laughter, goosebumps, a good meal, sunlight on your skin—as a form of orgasm. Let your body react. Let yourself sigh, moan, or smile without apology. Train your nervous system to recognize pleasure everywhere, not just in the bedroom.

> **Spicy Add-On:** Take this embodied experience all the way into ceremony. After edging together, choose a deliberate "peak" moment—set a timer, light a candle, or speak aloud, *"Now."* When the peak comes, let it be conscious and devotional: Moan their name, shout your own, or dedicate the convergence of sensation to something bigger—your healing, your relationship, your future creation. End by lying together in silence, feeling how the energy still lingers as sacred residue.

CHAPTER 14

DEVOTION BEYOND OBEDIENCE

THE SOVEREIGNTY OF LOVE

There is a silent grief that haunts many lovers.

A quiet ache beneath the surface of the stories we tell ourselves about what romantic commitment should look like.

We're taught that devotion means sacrifice—that love requires denying any hunger that could "threaten" the container. If we truly love someone, we will shrink our desires, keep our longings quiet, and swallow the part that craves more.

As a woman, if you own your hunger, you are branded a slut. As a man, you're called immature or a player if you explore it. Either way, hunger becomes suspicious—something to be hidden or justified.

Once I cracked open my erotic body, *I became one with the hunger*. For more intimacy. More eroticism. More *aliveness.*

That hunger was never about replacing anyone. It was about the truth of who I am.

For that, I've been called names—slut, whore, insatiable. At first, the words landed like blows, meant to put me in my place. Until one day, someone whispered "slut" in bed—and instead of shame, my body surged awake. My nipples tightened, my pussy pulsed to life, and I realized it wasn't the word itself that hurt. It was the meaning I'd let become tethered to it.

The truth was simpler: I wasn't broken. I was *alive*.

MISTAKING CONTROL FOR CARE

I once gave a Dominant the authority over who I could and could not play with. A power I'd never even given my husband.

We called it an experiment—a way to explore a deeper layer of trust and authority. I thought it might feel good to surrender that decision-making power, and to let Someone Else carry it.

What we were playing with was *ownership*—a dynamic that, for many people in D/s relationships, is deeply charged and sacred. For some, it's about structure and discipline, and yes, control. For others, it's about devotion, a feeling of protection, or of care. For many, it's all of the above—woven together with erotic tension and primal hunger.

At its highest, it can be medicine.

But here's what's not often talked about:

The desire for ownership—from either side of the "slash"—often arises from the fear of abandonment. From wounding or energetic entanglement. And when you understand that, everything shifts. You begin to see ownership as a longing for consistency and for holding. That's what I thought I was agreeing to. A space where I could set down the constant burden of deciding and containing and self-managing. Where His authority would be a form of care. Where my surrender would let me rest.

But real sovereignty means remembering *you never actually hand yourself over*. You can always take your power back.

Instead of meeting me in that sacred responsibility, He used the authority to shield His own insecurities. He began to limit my connections—not for my well-being, but to soothe His fear of comparison, His fear of not being enough, and, no doubt, other fears He never shared or wasn't even consciously aware of.

The rupture came when He denied me the chance to rope-bottom for a trusted friend, even though only months earlier He had asked for the exact same experience with a new woman. His desires were allowed; mine were restricted.

It wasn't the decision that ended us. It was the clarity. I was engaged in multiple relationships when we met, and that continued throughout our power exchange dynamic... until I gave that authority away. He only wanted me to engage with the parts of me that made Him feel safe.

And I had given Him the power to shut down the rest. So I had to take it back. Because devotion cannot be built on conditional sovereignty. My pleasure, my intimacy, and my relationships—they belonged to me.

The Dark Masculine in distortion limits from fear, mistaking control for care. The Dark Feminine in distortion abandons herself for safety, giving away power she was never meant to lose. That dynamic played out between us until I ended it.

Because true devotion is not obedience. True devotion is freedom chosen again and again.

REDEFINING FAITHFULNESS-IN-RELATIONSHIP

We've been taught that faithfulness-in-relationship means sexual or romantic exclusivity. But faithfulness isn't measured by how many people we touch or desire or love.

Faithfulness, to me, is:

- The courage to tell the truth.
- The commitment to show up as my full self, even when it's inconvenient.
- The refusal to abandon my erotic truth for someone else's comfort.
- The devotion to remain in alignment, even when it—and *I*—evolve.

I don't struggle with polyamory. I struggle with watching people abandon themselves to preserve a relationship. Faithfulness is not about what form or relationship style you commit to—it's about whether you remain faithful to yourself inside it. Because the moment you hide who you are, the love you're receiving isn't really yours at all—it's being given to the mask you put on, not the truth of your being.

ADORATION WITHOUT AGENDA

I remember slipping into the shower with Jimmy, the husband of a couple I often played with. Sometimes the three of us played, sometimes it was just he and I, and sometimes we played with the whole delicious constellation of sexy friends in our orbit.

That night, my body was still glowing with post-play buzz. As the hot water poured down, I began to gush with an open heart. I told him how much I enjoyed him; how grateful I was for the sweet connection.

His face tensed. He blurted, "You know I love my wife!"

I blinked, then laughed softly. Not mocking, just surprised. "I know. That's part of why I love being with you. It's how deeply you love her that makes me admire you even more."

I watched the tension melt from his shoulders. His body softened. Because what I was offering wasn't a bid for more. It was adoration—freely given, with nothing attached. No demand. No secret hook. Just *truth.*

I think we all need reminders sometimes. That expressing love doesn't mean "I want more." That devotion doesn't always mean "change something." Sometimes it just means *I see you. I value this. Thank you.*

This is what devotion looks like when it is sovereign. When it isn't trying to contort the other into meeting a hidden need. Just presence. Just love, with no agenda.

THE TRUTH ABOUT BEING A SUBMISSIVE

As an educator and leader in the kink community, I've seen this pattern play out again and again: Submissives are taught to hand over power completely. We glorify the idea of total surrender, of becoming property, and of letting a Dominant make every decision.

Submission doesn't mean abdicating responsibility for your life, for who you are outside of that submission, or outsourcing your growth to Someone Else. It's not about handing Another the impossible task of being your Healer or your Perfect Parent.

If you have a submissive identity in you, you *must* also know sovereignty. You must know yourself. You must know how to take your power back, which means ending the dynamic when it no longer serves you.

In the right hands, surrender becomes expansive. The Dark Feminine in her sovereignty yields not from weakness, but from power. She demands the Dominant meet her fully—to hold her without collapsing and guide her without diminishing her.

And the Dark Masculine in his sovereignty doesn't lead to control, but to elevate. He becomes the structure strong enough for her fire, the container steady enough for her storm.

Anything less is disempowerment. And devotion should never require that.

WHEN DEVOTION LOOKS LIKE FREEDOM

Commitment isn't about locking someone in. It's about what you choose when you could walk away—and choose not to.

For me, commitment means:

- I will look for ways to make you feel important to me.
- I will tell you the truth, even when it's hard.
- I will assume good intent when I'm triggered.

- I will be kind in conflict.
- I will take responsibility for my needs—not demanding them from you.
- I will support your joy, even if it challenges my comfort.

And I expect the same in return.

This is the deepest devotion I know: to love someone's truth more than their performance of love for me.

When we strip control away, something sacred emerges.

The Dark Feminine says: I will not shrink to be loved. The Dark Masculine says: **I will meet you with presence, not possession.**

Together, they create a field where love itself becomes a transmission.

But to arrive here, both must bring their wholeness—not just the polished parts. Because when you meet in sovereignty, you stop chasing love. You let love meet you.

CLOSING THE SCENE: THIS IS NOT EASY WORK

Let me be honest.

Everything I've written here may sound beautiful, empowering, even transcendent. But living it is hard. It asks you to let go of attachment. To sit in your own discomfort. To face rejection without self-abandonment. To love someone enough to let them walk away and love yourself enough not to collapse when they do.

This is not a path for the faint of heart. But it is *the path to love in its purest form.*

Love beyond control.

Devotion beyond obedience.

Two sovereigns meeting not with grasping hands, but with open palms.

That is where love becomes sacred ground.

EROTIC ALCHEMY IN PRACTICE: DEVOTION WITHOUT COLLAPSE

Embodiment

Say out loud a small truth you usually swallow—something as simple as "I'm tired," "I want more," or "I don't like that." Feel how your body reacts when you speak it into the room instead of keeping it inside. Notice if your chest loosens, if your jaw unclenches, or if your spine straightens. This is what coherence feels like in real time.

> **Spicy Add-On:** Do this while touching yourself—each time you moan, sigh, or whisper a truth, notice how your body responds. Let your arousal fuel your voice instead of silencing it.

Integration—Solo

Write down one truth you've been afraid to voice in a current relationship. Say it out loud to yourself in the mirror, to remind your body that it is safe to name what's real.

Notice how your breath, your voice, and your nervous system respond when your truth has air.

> **Spicy Add-On:** Find a mirror. As you watch yourself, strip your clothes down to whatever level of undress feels edgy. Then hold your own gaze and speak the truth to your reflection. Let the nakedness make the truth even bolder.

Integration—Partnered

Choose one small truth you've been holding back with someone—a longing, a limit, a desire. Share it with them without apology, without blaming, and without trying to manage their reaction. Your task is simply to speak it.

Spicy Add-On: Turn it into a ritual of erotic confession. One of you kneels or lies back while the other whispers truths into the air—secrets, desires, limits. The one receiving simply listens or offers acknowledgement like, "Thank you for sharing that with me," absorbing each one like an offering.

Then switch.

Integration (24-Hour Challenge)

Throughout the day, notice every time you edit yourself to avoid discomfort. When it happens, pause. Place a hand over your heart and whisper to yourself: *I will not abandon me.* Then, if it feels safe, let even a small piece of the truth be spoken aloud in that moment.

Spicy Add-On: If you're brave, share one of those truths with someone you trust—a friend, lover, or confidant who can hold it without judgment. This doesn't need to be the person the truth is *about*. The practice is in letting the truth leave your body and land in another's presence, without overexplaining or softening it.

CHAPTER 15

THE EDGE OF EDGES

PLAYING WITH THE RISKIEST KINKS

There is a threshold in erotic play where pleasure and pain blur, where control and surrender collapse into raw sensation. At that edge, the body and mind drop out, and what's left is pure signal. Some call it "subspace." Some call it trance. Some call it madness.

Every player finds their own way there. For some, that edge is fear play—the jolt of adrenaline as fight-or-flight meets surrender. For others, it's breath play—a dance with oxygen and control on the razor's edge between ecstasy and unconsciousness.

For me, one night, it came through something deceptively simple: a bottle of muscle rub, a stool, and a kinky crowd.

PUSSY ON FIRE

A sexy leather couple I trusted found me at a play party.

"Have you ever tried Kwan Loong Oil on your pussy?" they asked, half-grinning, half-warning.

I shook my head.

"It's like Tiger Balm with a grudge."

The masochist in me was intrigued. I'd done pussy torture before and liked most of it. The thought of heat against soft tissue, of fire licking at my most sensitive places, sounded… promising.

"One drop goes a long way. But it's a ride. Once you're on it, there's no going back."

They grinned as they explained, and even in my arousal I felt the warning underneath. Edge play should never be a surprise. It should be a plan.

I blushed with excitement, my heart racing. I had no idea how far I was about to be pushed.

I slipped my panties off, leaned back against a stool and spread my legs. The husband tapped one slick fingertip along my clit and at the threshold of my vagina. I blushed as they stared at me in anticipation…

At first: a faint warmth, like the brush of heat before a flame catches.

Then the switch flipped—within seconds, the sensation went from flash to blaze to full *firestorm*.

Intensity erupted from the core of me, spreading outward in pulsing waves, hot and cold at the same time, like molten ice. The air itself turned into fire. Every draft, every whisper of movement across my skin sent a fresh surge through my nerves.

All I could do was be present with the intensity. I literally sat on the edge of overwhelm.

They lifted me onto the stool, pinstripe mini kilt lifted, knees parted, fully exposed. A crowd gathered. I'd consented to being witnessed; that was part of my edge. The wife reached for a toy—a vibrating wand—pressing it against my already screaming flesh.

The vibration stacked on top of the heat until my whole system was signals—no narrative, no performance, just body.

I wasn't thinking. I wasn't deciding. I was only *a body reacting.*

Back arched. Fingers white-knuckled on wood. Thighs shaking with charge. I didn't need to manage it. The point was to be taken by it, and to stay present enough to ride it out.

Time fell out of the scene. I was no longer "me in a room." I was sensation moving through a human shape.

I'll never forget it. It was fucking incredible.

What made it safe wasn't luck—it was the thoughtful container. The Dark Masculine brought his structure (the quick negotiation, gloves, dose control, the toy, airflow, a clear stop). The Dark Feminine brought her raw power (my choice to ride the intensity without abandoning myself).

WHEN THE SCENE GOES SIDEWAYS

Different party. A night like many others—fetish wear, rig points, familiar faces. My wrists were cuffed high, my body long. The Top I was playing with had my favorite toys—floggers, canes, dragon's tongues, some mean custom rubber implements someone in our pack made. Around us, our friends played and fucked and cuddled and laughed.

I was ready. Or at least I thought I was. But from the first few strikes, my system said *nope*. It wasn't His technique or the tools. It was me.

Every hit landed *too* sharp, *too* loud—echoing inside like punishment. My body tensed in resistance. My marriage had been unraveling around that time, and apparently, so was something inside me.

I didn't safe word. Didn't ask to pause. Didn't speak up. I put on the *Let's do this* smirk and kept playing the high-capacity girl. Told Him we were still *green*.

We started up again. He saw through me. He stopped himself, stepped close, and checked in one more time with the kind of attunement a good Dominant or Top carries in his bones.

I cracked. "I don't know. Everything hurts differently. I just want to run."

He dropped the implements, moved straight to aftercare, and held me while my shame hit me harder than any cane ever could.

The scolding came later—clean, not cruel. He wasn't angry that I broke. He was pissed I didn't let him care for me sooner.

We did live demos together. Taught classes on rope, impact, soft skills, and squirting. Our scenes were often intense and public. I loved being the one who could take what He gave. I loved offering myself in that way.

Consent isn't paperwork. It's a living thread. If I hide where I am, I cut the thread we rely on when shit gets real.

I abandoned myself in that scene—too eager to be the "badass," too afraid to admit I was struggling. My distorted Dark Masculine wanted to muscle through; my distorted Dark Feminine wanted to be praised for holding it all. Both left me silent when what I really needed was to speak.

That night remapped something important: My edge isn't just in sensation. My edge is in telling the truth *while* the scene is happening.

The Dark Feminine in distortion overrides her own body to be "good." The Dark Masculine in distortion keeps swinging because the script says so.

In truth, this was one of my shadow patterns: performing strength instead of living my truth. I wanted to be the woman who could take anything, who never broke—but that wasn't power. That was me abandoning myself in the name of looking powerful.

In coherence, she names what's real; he adjusts the container. That's the whole game.

SIDEBAR: Edge Readiness Checks

- ***Before:*** *What state am I in? What states might show up (nonverbal, freeze, dissociation)? What are our reconnect signals?*
- ***During:*** *Who's tracking breath, eyes, muscle tone, temperature, words? What auto-stop ends the scene?*

- ***After:*** *What's the landing plan (touch, warmth, water, electrolytes, carbs, quiet, story)? Who checks in twenty-four hours later?*

WHY THE EDGE CALLS

The body has limits, but they're not fixed. They can be stretched, dissolved, and rewritten when we understand how to work with them. Extreme kink isn't just about how much you can take. It's about what opens when you go there. Edges reveal what our ordinary-self hides.

Extreme kinks tap into:

The Adrenaline High—Some people crave fear play, captivity scenes, or predicament bondage not because they want to suffer, but because the body's fight-or-flight response creates a rush of alertness and intensity. When curated consciously, that rush becomes a portal into pure aliveness.

The Neurological Surrender—When sensation goes past what the brain recognizes as normal, the thinking mind drops away. This can open the door to subspace, trance states, or altered consciousness—where instinct takes over, and the body begins responding from a deeper intelligence than thought.

The Pleasure/Pain Threshold—When arousal is high, the nervous system can alchemize pain into pleasure. The sting becomes a pulse of light. The whip becomes a kiss. What once overwhelmed now turns you on.

The Altered State of Submission—When you're no longer performing or trying to manage the experience, your most unguarded self emerges. Your nervous system opens. Your breath deepens. Emotions, memories, or desires you didn't know you were holding can come forward for release or reclamation.

At the edge, you find exactly what you want, what you fear, and what you're ready to release.

RISKY KINKS, CLEAN FRAMES—WAYS PEOPLE EXPLORE EDGES

Not all edges feel the same. Some take you to the edge of your body. Others take you to the edge of your psyche. What they all share is this: high stakes, deep trust, and the potential for radical transformation—if engaged with care. Conscious curiosity won't cut it. These practices demand self-awareness, skilled partners, and clear, grounded agreements. Below are some of the most intense—and illuminating—ways people explore their limits.

Breath Play—The Line Between Power and Peril

Air is power. The high of controlled oxygen deprivation can unlock altered states, heightened arousal, and deep surrender. If you play here, you need skill, signals, timing, and humility. The thrill is control; the risk is hubris. The coherent Dark Masculine must be forensic about safety: hand placement, timing windows, recovery signs. No bravado.

Sensory Edge Play—Rewiring Perception Through the Body

Some kinks bypass pain entirely and drop you into altered states through sensation alone. These practices recalibrate your nervous system, slowing the world down or flooding it with information. Electro, temperature, deprivation/overload. These don't require pain to alter state; they require precision. Treat them like instruments rather than stunts.

Predicament & Fear Play—Psychological Edges

Sometimes the deepest edge isn't physical—it's mental. Predicament play traps you between impossible choices. Fear play awakens the body's primal responses in a container of safety. **That paradox is the charge**. Do this with people who can co-regulate you—not ones who just excite you.

Forced Orgasms & Endurance Play—Broken Open by Pleasure

Too much pleasure can overwhelm the body, but that overwhelm can also be the doorway. When pushed past the usual limits, people may shake, cry, laugh, or even collapse. What's really happening is that the protective layers around receiving begin to give way.

Forced orgasm and endurance play aren't about numbers or performance. They're about how the nervous system responds when stimulation continues past the point of comfort or control. In these scenes, the measure isn't "how many peaks" but whether the bottom feels safe and held as their defenses dissolve.

That's why these dynamics aren't ego contests. They are crafts—requiring skill, pacing, and attunement. The deeper the edge, the more important it is that the Top's hands are clean, steady, and precise.

If you're called to explore these edges, don't do it alone. Find partners who read your breath, your eyes, and your nervous system, not just your words.

RETURNING FROM THE FIRE—INTEGRATION

After that Kwan Loong Oil scene—after the ache and the adrenaline, the vibrator, and the surrender—I was still floating.

My body hummed with the aftershock of everything it had just held. I wasn't quite *all there*, but I wasn't gone either. Suspended in a liminal space edge players know well: not pain, not pleasure… just open.

That's when they came for me. S&J. A couple I'd been dating for years—familiar, safe, attuned. They took my hand and led me to a spanking bench, my body still reverberating. She nestled behind me, cradling my heart and head, anchoring me. He knelt between my legs, mouth soft, tongue offering slow, tender worship to delicate skin still buzzing from impact.

No escalation. No new challenge. Just a slow descent back into the body.

Pleasure-as-aftercare is underrated medicine: not more intensity, but integration—breath, eye contact, water, salt, something sweet, warmth; words only when they return. Dark Masculine closes the ritual; Dark Feminine receives until the system says "home."

You can go to the edge. If you want alchemy, you must also return.

STAYING SAFE AT THE EDGE

When you're about to step into edge play, don't just talk about what you *want to do*—talk about the states you might drop into. If you know you sometimes go quiet or nonverbal, name that ahead of time and agree on a clear signal you can still give if you need the scene to pause or stop.

Decide together what will stop the scene, no matter what. You don't need to prove how tough you are by muscling through. Sometimes the bravest thing you can do is know where "enough" really lives.

Remember that consent isn't locked in at the beginning—it shifts. A full-body yes at the start of a scene can become a shaky maybe halfway through. Give yourselves permission to pause, to re-check, and to listen to what's real in the moment.

Plan your landing before you ever take off. Aftercare isn't optional—it's how your nervous system comes back, how trust gets sealed, and how the whole thing becomes integration instead of just intensity.

If you're the one holding the scene, track the human in front of you more than the scene in your head. Notice their breath, the look in their eyes, the way their body is holding tension. Believe what you see, not just what they say.

And if you're the one surrendering, know this: using a safe word doesn't make you weak. It means you're listening to your body. It means you trust yourself. That trust is the strongest power you can bring into a scene.

CLOSING THE SCENE: THE EDGE EXISTS FOR A REASON

Some people never touch these edges. Others live at them.

But edge isn't about danger; it's about discernment—knowing where your line lives, deciding who gets to meet you there, and who can bring you back with your name still in your mouth.

Intensity is easy to find. Discernment is the art—the ability to read the moment, feel what's true, and know when to press forward and when to pull back.

The mastery is playing close to the flame—with the Dark Feminine free to devour, and the Dark Masculine stalwart enough to hold—without either of you disappearing.

EROTIC ALCHEMY IN PRACTICE: PLAYING AT THE THRESHOLD

Embodiment

Think of a time when you wanted to challenge your own edge—whether in kink, sport, or another risk. Let the memory land in your body then notice the physical sensations. Did your heart race? Did your breath catch? Did you find yourself leaning forward? Place your hands on your body and breathe into that set of sensations, that charge. Let yourself feel how alive the edge makes you.

> **Spicy Add-On:** While self-pleasuring, take yourself to a sensory edge—that might look like edging toward climax then pausing, or adding a sensation (ice, heat, a rougher grip). When the intensity builds, breathe with it. Instead of rushing through or avoiding the feeling, let your breath steady you so you can actually feel the heat, the ache, the pulse of sensation moving through your body.

Integration—Solo

Pick a low-stakes "edge"—colder shower, one more rep at the gym, saying something bold out loud. As you approach that edge, notice when your body wants to stop. Stay with it a few breaths longer. Track how the Dark Feminine shows up in the hunger for more, and how the Dark Masculine shows up in the structure that steadies you.

> **Spicy Add-On:** Use self-pleasure as the playground. Edge yourself: Bring arousal close to climax, then hold yourself there. Instead of releasing right away, stay

with the heightened sensation—notice the pulse, the vibration, the reaching in your body. Breathe into all of it and let yourself feel how the experience expands when you don't rush to finish. Repeat this a few times, and track how power builds when you hold yourself at that edge.

Integration—Partnered

With a trusted partner or friend, create a simple, negotiated edge scene. It doesn't need to be extreme—try impact play, tickling, or restraint with scarves. Agree on how you'll communicate during the scene, and on a clear stop. One person plays with giving intensity with precision and presence, the other practices receiving and tracking their body's response.

Swap roles if you choose.

Afterward, debrief together.

> **Spicy Add-On:** Add a layer of risk—blindfold the receiver, add music, or invite an audience of one trusted friend to watch. Notice how the energy spikes when you add just one more layer of the unknown.

PART FIVE: THE FINAL EDGE

PLEASURE AS SPIRITUAL MASTERY

BEFORE YOU TURN THE PAGE...

These books aren't just stories I tell. They're *edges* I live.

Every chapter I write becomes a threshold I walk in real time—an initiation that demands more depth, more truth, and more surrender from me. I don't write *about* transformation. I write *through* it. And each time I do, I become more of who I came here to be.

Forbidden Alchemy took me to one of my deepest edges yet—the place where shame and desire collided. Where need became choice. Where the edge itself disappeared altogether...

I wrote the first fifteen chapters from the rawest truth I had access to. And then I paused. I knew the book wasn't complete, but the final chapter hadn't revealed itself yet. It wasn't one I could plan.

So I turned inward. I got still. I listened.

An idea surfaced. A stretch-goal of erotic mastery.

At that point in my journey, I was already fluent in many kinds of orgasms.

- Physical orgasms, from clitoral or penetrative touch.
- Fantasy orgasms, where my climax depended on a story I played in my head.

- Energetic orgasms, where a lover's touch, presence, or even their *field* alone sent waves through my body.
- Kundalini orgasms, cultivated through breath and energy practice until the current surged like fire through my body.

But here's the difference: In all of those, something else was the spark—touch, fantasy, another's energy, or the rising current of built Kundalini. Even if those orgasms didn't start from my genitals, they still came from stimulation, from effort, or from cultivation of some kind.

I wanted something different. I didn't want to be triggered from the outside, or even from the effort of building energy within. I wanted to summon orgasm through sheer choice. A climax born of simple command, erupting because I willed it. Because my body was that coherent. That alive, and free.

That became the goal. I imagined I'd have to train for it—slow, solo practice over time.

The Universe had other plans. As it always does when I ask and then surrender, it delivered. Not in the way I expected, but in a way so exact, so cellular, that it rewired my body before my mind even realized what had changed.

And that's what brings us here.

The chapter you're about to read is the culmination of that unfolding. A story I didn't know was still being written. A full-circle answer to a prayer I almost forgot I asked.

This is the moment when the edge dissolves. When the Dark Feminine's surrender becomes the Dark Masculine's initiation. When chaos and order meet in the same body. When pleasure itself becomes the current of creation.

Because the final mastery was never about waiting for someone else to ignite me. It was about becoming the spark.

This chapter is that ignition.

CHAPTER 16

THE SACRED RETURN

DEVOTION AS INTEGRATION

This chapter is the final threshold. Not because it closes the story, but because it dissolves the illusion that anything was ever separate, and reminds us that pleasure, pain, innocence, and power are all part of the same flame.

When we stop running from ourselves—when we allow our deepest hungers and hidden shadows to be celebrated—we come home. Not to an ending. But to a full-bodied beginning.

MY DIVINE PRIMAL EMERGENCE

It wasn't planned. It rarely is when the divine arrives.

After over a year of profound interactions with Daniel, my Daddy Dom—a man whose presence had become deeply healing and precision-attuned—something unexpected happened.

We'd already shared beautiful, layered experiences, each one allowing my inner Baby Girl to heal and joyfully blossom.

But we had a series of encounters, nearly back-to-back, that broke everything open.

We usually met twice a month—once for lunch and once for a sexy date. For my birthday, He'd curated a decadent day and night together: a hotel suite, port-finished rye, a Harley ride and dinner at a winery, a sunset soak in the hot tub, and a long night of lovemaking that shifted from slow, devotional touch into a gloriously dirty marathon. For the first time, we stayed in the same space overnight, light sleepers side by side, choosing to rest in the same room.

The date was delicious. And just like that first time I said *Daddy* aloud, it shifted something between us.

After the date, we messaged each other about how attunement makes us better lovers and parents, and better citizens of the world. The debrief of the date, and the conversation thread, were electric. We couldn't help ourselves. We scheduled another date only ten days later—a deviation from our usual rhythm.

That afternoon, I wore lingerie I knew He'd love. During play, He held me down with *His steady, playful strength* and teased:

"See? This is what happens when you're just so sexy." His voice was breathy. "When you wear sexy things like this for Me, this is what you get… Daddy's full attention and appreciation."

I laughed out loud, fully in my body. Turned on and safe. His tone wasn't entitled or possessive. It was adoring and anchored and reverent. It carried just enough of a playful, loving edge—"This pleasure is *your* fault…"—that ignited a score of my kinks at once: focused attention, restraint, incest/power imbalance fantasy, and the thrill of being prized by the coherent Dark Masculine.

Then He said something else. "You know… this, what we've got right here, is the stuff most people don't even know to fantasize about. This is something special. I love my sexy Baby Girl Goddess…"

He'd been calling me that for months. I adored the juxtaposition—*baby girl* and *goddess*—but until that moment, I hadn't realized why it landed so deeply.

***SIDEBAR: Why I Capitalized* Baby Girl**

In kink shorthand, Daddy Dom/baby girl dynamics are often written as DD/bg. The lowercase bg is a common way to denote the submissive role in writing, but that designation is not a statement of value. In these pages you'll see me refer to both Daddy and Baby Girl in caps. This is intentional. My Baby Girl isn't "less than." She is not a diminished part of me, nor a fragment of smallness. She is a whole, sovereign aspect—erotic, playful, tender, and potent. She is the frequency I choose to embody inside this polarity, not a symbol of inferiority. I capitalize Baby Girl *because she is an archetypal presence within me. A goddess in pigtails. Another current of my divine erotic nature. To me, the all-caps are a gesture of reverence—honoring her as equal, sacred, and exalted in the dynamic Daniel and I co-create.*

Daniel continued to speak—more praise, more naming of my uniqueness, more love for being my Daddy and feeling *made for me*—that's when something inside me shifted. The little girl I thought had integrated that night with Scott fully rose to the surface. Again. The part of me who had longed to be adored by a loving masculine finally heard the words she'd waited her whole life to hear.

And suddenly, there was no divide between her and me anymore. We were merged. Wanted. Naughty. Worshipped. Beloved.

I don't want to make this sound like my journey was always "pure." I had spent years performing devotion to be loved rather than letting devotion rise authentically. That was my distorted Dark Feminine at work—mistaking self-abandonment for sacred surrender. This time was different because I brought all of me, even the parts I used to exile.

And it wasn't just His cock or His words that unlocked me. It was His *frequency*—steady, attuned, unguarded. His body and breath said: *You are not too much. You are welcome here.*

This wasn't just play. This was medicine.

A FUSION OF SELVES

Days later, we met again. A third date in two weeks—unheard of for us. This time, something entirely new arrived. I had met my Baby Girl countless times. I had felt my Goddess before. I had called my ancestors into the room. But never had they all fused.

As He praised me more, something clicked into place. My body started vibrating with a faster frequency. My Goddess Self descended like lightning, all-powerful. My Baby Girl rose with her innocence intact. They folded into one another.

Then other past selves rose. Ancestors stirred.

Every denied, hidden, or fragmented version of me surfaced. And one by one, through His full presence and authentic love, each was seen and integrated.

I cried. I came. I laughed. I surrendered. A circuit formed—heart to heart, heart to cock, cock to pussy, pussy back to heart—over and over.

I'd read about this in tantra books. Felt hints of it before. But this was the first time every part of me—Baby Girl. Goddess. Lover. Priestess. Beast—existed in the same room, fused, whole, and sovereign.

That fusion was the first taste of what I now call **the Divine Primal**—the part of us that isn't split between chaos and order, or innocence and power. It's **the current that holds it all together, not as opposites but as one complete field.** At that moment, I wasn't switching between roles or archetypes. I was simply myself, unfragmented.

And in that moment, I knew: Power and innocence aren't opposites. Hunger and holiness can live in the same breath.

The Dark Feminine pulsed beneath it all—a throne reclaimed. The Dark Masculine met her—grounded and loving—not to tame, but to partner. To hold steady while she burned and transformed.

For the first time in my life, I wasn't trying to prove anything. I wasn't performing. I wasn't withholding. I was simply... *whole*.

Afterward, when I asked Him what He had felt as He was saying those things, He couldn't even remember His own words. He said, "When I touch and kiss your neck, and your soft cheek is next to mine, and I can hear your pleasure and feel you open to Me… it's all on autopilot. Touching what needs to be touched, kissing what needs to be kissed, saying what needs to be said."

He became the channel for my upleveling.

He rose as I did.

THE SOVEREIGN ORGASM

A few mornings later, during my morning meditation, I climaxed at will—no touch, no fantasy, no external spark. Just presence, desire, and the choice to say: now.

The decision itself was the ignition. And it was instantaneous because I was simply not allowing any internal resistance to stop it.

My body became the temple. My breath, the prayer. And my orgasm… the answer.

This was the edge I had set out to meet—the mastery I had only imagined. And reaching it, I realized: The point was never just the orgasm itself. It was what the orgasm revealed—that devotion and unconditional self-love is the real alchemy. That every peak is sacred only if it fuses you back into yourself.

And devotion is what makes that fusion possible. Devotion to myself. Devotion in union. Devotion as the alchemy.

CLOSING THE SCENE: DEVOTION IS THE ALCHEMY

With Daniel, this devotion wasn't fairy tale love. It wasn't about forever. It was about presence—the kind built through every yes, every truth, every unarmored meeting.

This is Sacred Union. Sovereignty with surrender. Choice without control. Devotion without domestication.

For years, I had whispered affirmations to my inner child alone. Held her through pain. Loved her in secret. But sometimes true integration requires a witness—not to complete us, but to seal the truth in the body like *kintsugi*—veins of gold running through the once-shattered places.

Erotic alchemy is this same process: It resurrects what was forgotten, fuses what was fractured, and makes the cracks themselves the source of radiance.

It returns us to the power that was always ours. Whole. Radiant. Unmistakably divine.

Your pleasure is your alchemical portal. Your desire is the map.

You were never at the mercy of your pleasure—you were always its master.

Welcome home.

EROTIC ALCHEMY IN PRACTICE: DEVOTION AS INTEGRATION

Embodiment

Take a quiet moment and place your hand over your heart. Breathe until you feel your chest rise and fall with steadiness. Recall a time when you felt fractured—when different parts of you (child, lover, achiever, caretaker) felt separate or even at odds. Notice how your body responds to that memory.

Then bring to mind a time when you felt whole—everything in you woven together. Feel the difference in your breath, your shoulders, your belly. This is the work of integration: not erasing the parts but letting them belong in the same body.

> **Spicy Add-On:** Touch yourself in two contrasting ways at once—one hand slow and tender, the other firmer or rougher. Imagine each hand as a different part of you (child, lover, caretaker, rebel). Notice what happens when those parts are felt together instead of apart.

Integration—Solo

Choose one way to *devote to yourself* today. It could be a slow bath, an unhurried meal, a walk in nature, or intentional self-praise. Whatever you choose, let the act become ritual. Speak to yourself as you would a beloved: *I am here. I am whole. I am sacred.* Let this devotion land in your body as self-honoring truth rather than performance.

> **Spicy Add-On:** During self-pleasure, whisper those same words aloud to yourself—"I am here. I am whole. I am

sacred." Let arousal become the amplifier of devotion, each wave reinforcing the truth that no part of you is left out.

Integration—Partnered (or Community)

Invite someone you trust into a simple ritual of witnessing. Stand or sit across from each other. Take turns speaking one truth about yourself you are reclaiming: *I am beautiful. I am sovereign. I am erotic. I am whole.* The other person's role is not to respond, but to hold steady presence and eye contact.

Notice what it feels like to be received without needing to shrink, prove, or explain.

> **Spicy Add-On:** Layer erotic energy into the ritual. While one person speaks their truths, the other offers slow, deliberate touch—holding a hand, tracing a shoulder, or stroking skin reverently. Let the physical contact anchor the words into the body.

Integration (24-Hour Challenge)

For the next day, track the moments when different "selves" rise up—your worker, your lover, your parent, your dreamer. Each time, pause to name them: "Ah, here's my caretaker." "Here's my seductress." Then remind yourself: *All of them are me.* Practice carrying them together instead of splitting them apart.

> **Spicy Add-On:** Pick one of those selves you've been most likely to exile (your slut, your boss, your brat, your teacher). For one day, deliberately eroticize them—let them guide how you dress, flirt, self-touch, or speak. Treat their presence not as something to hide, but as part of your turn-on.

ONE FINAL INVITATION

You were never meant to settle. Never meant to shrink. Never meant to sacrifice yourself just to belong.

This book was never about learning to tolerate your edges—it was about remembering you were born to meet them, dissolve them, and create beyond them.

You are the alchemist. The sovereign. The living flame of your own desire.

The last page of this book is written. But the alchemy? That begins with you.

Let your desire write the next chapter. Let your edges become your compass.

You are the edge.

ACKNOWLEDGMENTS

To Daniel—one of my deepest mirrors of the Dark Masculine. Thank you for your steadiness, your precision, and your presence. Your devotion and love became medicine that allowed me to emerge the most whole I've ever been.

To the lovers who have walked with me—you taught me through delight and through rupture, through passion and through pain. Each of you revealed a facet of my erotic self I could not have uncovered alone. Your bodies, your truths, your edges—all of it has been part of my expansion.

To Katie—mentor, ally, and vision-holder. You saw the empire I was building before I could name it myself, and helped me step into it with both feet.

To my kinky pack—the wild circle of friends who walked beside me in these years of discovery. We once called ourselves The Tribe, but what we really were was a constellation of mirrors. By contrast and by complement, you helped me grow into the woman and leader I am today. Your courage, playfulness, and hunger shaped every page of this book.

To my editor and publishing team—thank you for helping me bring this taboo medicine into form with clarity and courage.

And to every reader who dares to turn these pages—you are the continuation of this spell.

NEXT STEPS

This book is not the end—it's an initiation.

Join me inside Life Turned On for the next edge, the next desire, the next remembering.

Find me at sharonmariescott.com or subscribe to my Substack at sharonmariescott.substack.com for writing, practices, and transmissions straight from the edge of desire.

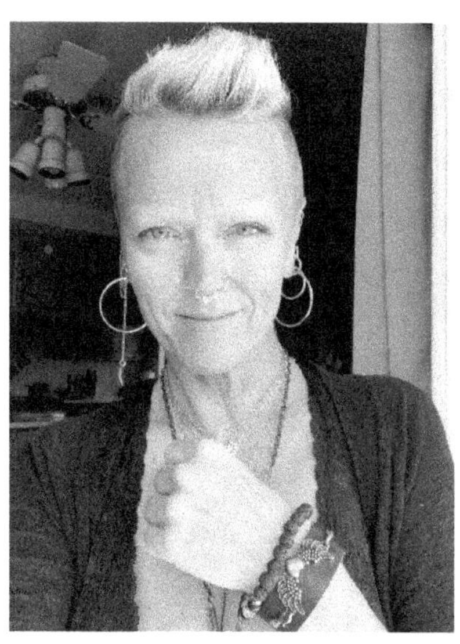

ABOUT THE AUTHOR

Sharon Marie Scott is a High Alchemist, storyteller, and founder of Life Turned On, a living temple devoted to desire, devotion, and spiritual mastery. Her work bridges the erotic and the divine, guiding self-led high-achievers, edge-players, and spiritual adventurers to remember their pleasure as sacred and their sovereignty as power.

For more than a decade, Sharon immersed herself in alternative lifestyles and sacred erotic practices—exploring kink, BDSM, tantra, open relating, sex-positive communities, and queerness as living laboratories for transformation. These experiences, combined with her own initiations into the sacred erotic mysteries, inform the depth and authenticity of her work today.

Forbidden Alchemy: Transmuting Taboo into Erotic Medicine is the first release in her Hieros Codex series. *Flesh & Flame: Pleasure as the Portal to Divine Mastery* is due out in February

2026. These works reimagine the path of ascension through desire, union, and ecstatic embodiment.

A veteran storyteller, Sharon spent more than two decades in the worlds of comics, video games, screenwriting, and fiction before turning her lens inward. Today, she speaks, inspires, and writes about sacred pleasure as the ultimate frontier of freedom.

For more great books from Empower Press
Visit Books.GracePointPublishing.com

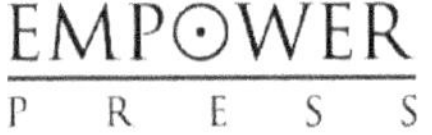

If you enjoyed reading *Forbidden Alchemy,* and purchased it through an online retailer, please return to the site and write a review to help others find the book.

www.ingramcontent.com/pod-product-compliance
Lightning Source LLC
LaVergne TN
LVHW010656110826
845149LV00014B/3119

9781966346678